BLOOD TYPE O POSITIVE DIET COOKBOOK

Complete Guide for Optimal Health and Wellness Eating With Heart Healthy Nutritious Recipes Tailored to Your Type

DETAILED CONTENTS

CHAPTER 1 INTRODUCTION

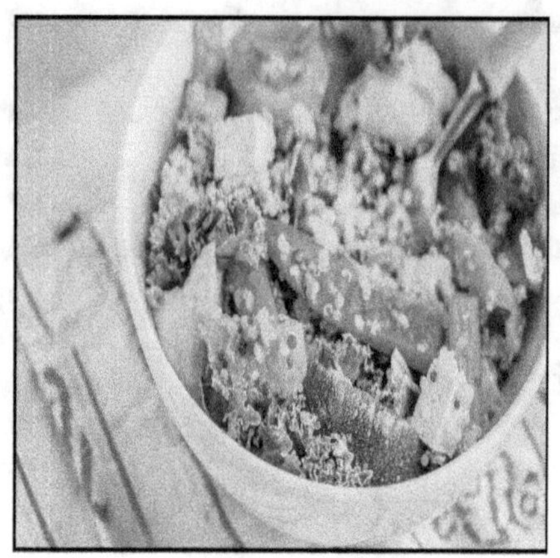

Welcome to the culinary journey made just for lively individuals with Blood Type O Positive! In this cookbook, you'll embark on a flavorful journey designed to not only satisfy your taste senses but also fuel your specific nutritional needs.

Picture this: A dining experience in which each dish is expertly prepared to meet the needs of your Blood Type O Positive. As you turn the pages, you'll discover a world of delicious dishes that celebrate the rich tapestry of flavors while encouraging overall health.

Join us as we reveal the secrets of a diet tailored to your blood type, featuring a symphony of proteins, fruits, vegetables, and grains precisely choreographed to boost your vitality. Whether you're a seasoned chef or a newbie in the kitchen, this cookbook will help you create delicious meals that are tailored to your specific dietary needs.

Each recipe is more than just a collection of ingredients; it's a culinary hug intended to improve your dining experience. So, put on your apron, sharpen your knives, and prepare to savor the delectable combination of health and taste.

Allow this cookbook to lead you in changing your kitchen into a haven where every meal is not only a feast for the senses, but also a tribute to the special needs of Blood Type O Positives. Welcome to the Blood Type O Positive Diet Cookbook, where nourishment and enjoyment dwell in perfect harmony!

UNDERSTANDING BLOOD TYPE O POSITIVE

Unlock the secrets of your vitality with "Understanding Blood Type O Positive" - a compelling inquiry that goes beneath the surface.

In this informative trip, we will uncover the distinct qualities that identify people with Blood Type O Positive, revealing insights into the essence of their genetic makeup. Discover why your body thrives on a specific combination of nutrients, and how this understanding can be the key to realising your full potential.

Dive into the world of personalised nutrition, where every food choice contributes to your overall health. Discover why some meals are compatible with your blood type, and how these choices affect your energy levels, metabolism, and overall health.

However, it is more than just knowing what to eat; it is also important to understand why. We dig deeper into the research, investigating the links between blood type and optimal nutrition. With this insight, you'll be able to make informed decisions that resonate with your body, sustaining it in ways that are unique to you.

Prepare for a riveting voyage of self-discovery and empowerment. "Understanding Blood Type O Positive" is more than a chapter; it's a revelation that will change the way you see your health. Let's explore the connection between your blood type and a fulfilling life.

BENEFITS OF FOLLOWING A BLOOD TYPE O POSITIVE DIET

1. Enhanced Energy Levels: Tailoring your diet to your blood type promotes a healthy relationship with food, resulting in sustained energy throughout the day.
2. Optimized Metabolism: Eat a diet that matches your blood type, which promotes efficient metabolism and aids in weight management.
3. Improved Digestion: Say goodbye to digestive discomfort by matching your dietary choices to your blood type, creating a gut-friendly environment.
4. Muscle Preservation: The Blood Type O Positive Diet's protein-rich focus promotes muscle preservation and development, making it ideal for an active lifestyle.
5. Enhanced Immune Function: Feed your body foods that are compatible with your blood type, which may boost immune function and resilience to illness.
6. Balanced Nutrient Intake: With a diet developed specifically for Blood Type O Positive, you can achieve a well-rounded nutritional profile while still getting the vital vitamins and minerals your body requires.
7. Potential Weight Loss Support: Tailoring your meals to your blood type may help you lose weight by facilitating proper digestion and metabolism.
8. Cognitive Clarity: Maintain mental sharpness by feeding your brain the nutrition it requires with a diet that is appropriate for your Blood Type O Positive.
9. Overall Well-Being: Experience the holistic advantages of a diet that matches your genetic composition, promoting balance, vitality, and well-being.

DIETARY GUIDELINES FOR BLOOD TYPE O POSITIVE

1. Protein-rich foods include lean meats like beef, lamb, and venison, as well as fowl like chicken and turkey.
   Prioritize seafood, particularly those high in omega-3 fatty acids, such as salmon and cod.
2. Recommended Vegetables and Fruits: Include nutrient-dense veggies like spinach, kale, and broccoli.

Choose antioxidant-rich fruits such as berries, cherries, and plums.

3. Whole Grains and Legumes: Include quinoa, rice, lentils, and navy beans.
   Limit or avoid wheat-based goods and specific legumes.

4. Dairy and Eggs: Consume dairy items such as yogurt and feta cheese in moderation.
   Incorporate eggs as a protein source, but keep them in balance.

CHAPTER 2: BREAKFAST RECIPES

Omelette with Spinach and Turkey:

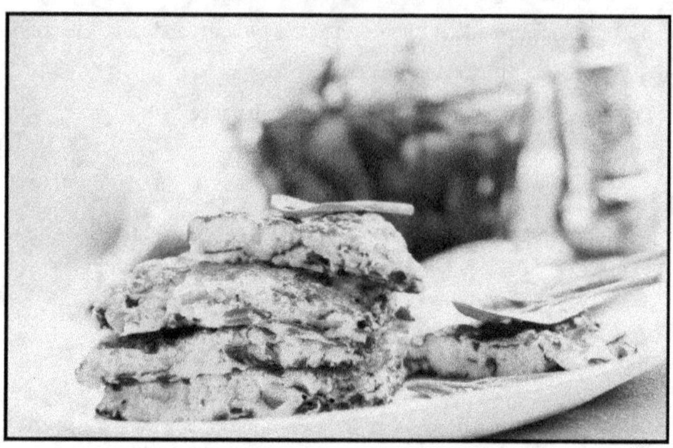

Ingredients:

- 3 large eggs (preferably organic)
- 1/2 cup cooked turkey, diced
- 1 cup fresh spinach, chopped
- 1/4 cup red bell pepper, finely chopped
- 1/4 cup onion, finely chopped
- 1 clove garlic, minced
- 1 tablespoon olive oil
- Salt and pepper to taste

Instructions:

1. In a bowl, beat the eggs until well combined. Season with salt and pepper according to your taste preferences.
2. Heat olive oil in a non-stick skillet over medium heat.
3. Add chopped onion and garlic to the skillet, sauté until softened.
4. Add diced turkey to the skillet and cook until it's slightly browned.

5. Toss in the chopped spinach and red bell pepper, stirring until the spinach wilts and the bell pepper is tender.

6. Pour the beaten eggs over the turkey and vegetable mixture in the skillet.

7. Allow the eggs to set around the edges. Gently lift the edges with a spatula, allowing the uncooked eggs to flow underneath.

8. When the omelette is mostly set but still slightly runny on top, fold it in half using the spatula.

9. Cook for an additional minute or until the eggs are fully cooked through.

10. Slide the omelette onto a plate, and serve immediately.

Quinoa Breakfast Bowl:

Ingredients:

- 1 cup cooked quinoa
- 1/2 cup almond milk (or any preferred milk)
- 1 tablespoon honey or maple syrup
- 1/2 teaspoon vanilla extract
- 1/2 cup fresh mixed berries (blueberries, strawberries, raspberries)
- 1 medium banana, sliced
- 1 tablespoon chia seeds
- 1 tablespoon chopped nuts (e.g., almonds, walnuts)
- Greek yogurt (optional, for topping)

Instructions:

1. In a saucepan, heat the almond milk over medium heat until warm but not boiling.

2. Stir in the honey or maple syrup and vanilla extract, ensuring they are well combined.

3. Add the cooked quinoa to the saucepan and stir to coat the quinoa with the sweetened almond milk mixture. Heat for a few minutes until warmed through.

4. Remove the quinoa mixture from heat and transfer it to a breakfast bowl.

5. Top the quinoa with mixed berries, banana slices, chia seeds, and chopped nuts.

6. If desired, add a dollop of Greek yogurt on top for extra creaminess.

7. Drizzle with additional honey or maple syrup for sweetness, if desired.

8. Mix all the ingredients in the bowl just before eating to combine flavors.

Turkey and Avocado Wrap:

Ingredients:

- 1 large whole-grain or spinach tortilla
- 4 ounces cooked turkey breast, thinly sliced
- 1/2 avocado, sliced
- 1/4 cup cherry tomatoes, halved
- 1/4 cup cucumber, thinly sliced
- 2 tablespoons Greek yogurt or hummus
- 1 tablespoon Dijon mustard (optional)
- Fresh lettuce leaves
- Salt and pepper to taste

Instructions:

1. Lay the tortilla flat on a clean surface or plate.

2. In the center of the tortilla, spread a layer of Greek yogurt or hummus, leaving about an inch border around the edges.

3. Place the thinly sliced turkey evenly over the yogurt or hummus layer.

4. Arrange avocado slices, cherry tomatoes, and cucumber on top of the turkey.

5. If desired, add Dijon mustard for an extra kick.

6. Season with salt and pepper to taste.

7. Place fresh lettuce leaves over the ingredients.

8. Fold in the sides of the tortilla and then roll it up tightly from the bottom, creating a wrap.

9. Cut the wrap in half diagonally for easier handling, if preferred.

10. Serve immediately, or wrap in parchment paper for an on-the-go meal.

Greek Yogurt Parfait:

Ingredients:

- 1 cup Greek yogurt (plain or flavored)
- 1/2 cup granola
- 1/2 cup mixed berries (strawberries, blueberries, raspberries)
- 1 tablespoon honey or maple syrup
- 1/4 cup chopped nuts (e.g., almonds, walnuts)
- 1/2 teaspoon vanilla extract (optional)

Instructions:

1. In a glass or a bowl, start by layering a spoonful of Greek yogurt at the bottom.
2. Sprinkle a layer of granola over the yogurt.
3. Add a layer of mixed berries on top of the granola.
4. Drizzle a bit of honey or maple syrup over the berries.
5. Repeat the layers until you reach the top of the glass or bowl.
6. If desired, sprinkle chopped nuts over the final layer for added crunch.
7. Optionally, add a touch of vanilla extract to the Greek yogurt for extra flavor.
8. Repeat the layering process if preparing multiple servings.
9. Serve immediately, or refrigerate until ready to eat.
10. Use a long spoon to reach all the layers while enjoying the parfait.

Salmon and Avocado Toast:

Ingredients:

- 2 slices whole-grain bread or your preferred bread
- 4 ounces smoked salmon
- 1 ripe avocado, sliced
- 1 tablespoon cream cheese or Greek yogurt
- 1 tablespoon capers (optional)
- Fresh dill or chives for garnish
- Lemon wedges for serving

- Salt and pepper to taste

Instructions:

1. Toast the slices of bread to your preferred level of crispiness.
2. Spread a thin layer of cream cheese or Greek yogurt on each slice of toast.
3. Lay slices of smoked salmon over the cream cheese or yogurt.
4. Place avocado slices on top of the salmon.
5. If using, sprinkle capers evenly over the avocado.
6. Season with salt and pepper to taste.
7. Garnish with fresh dill or chives for added flavor and visual appeal.
8. Squeeze a bit of lemon juice over the top for a zesty finish.
9. Serve the Salmon and Avocado Toast immediately.
10. Enjoy this delicious and nutritious open-faced sandwich as a satisfying breakfast or brunch option.

Smoothie with Kale and Pineapple:

Ingredients:

- 1 cup kale leaves, stems removed and chopped
- 1 cup fresh or frozen pineapple chunks
- 1 ripe banana
- 1/2 cup Greek yogurt
- 1/2 cup coconut water or water
- 1 tablespoon chia seeds (optional)
- Ice cubes (if not using frozen pineapple)
- Honey or maple syrup to taste (optional)

Instructions:

1. Place the kale, pineapple chunks, banana, Greek yogurt, and chia seeds (if using) in a blender.
2. Add coconut water or water to the blender.
3. If you prefer a sweeter smoothie, you can add honey or maple syrup at this stage.

4. Blend the ingredients on high speed until smooth and creamy. If the consistency is too thick, you can add more liquid.

5. If using fresh pineapple, add a handful of ice cubes and blend again until the smoothie reaches your desired consistency.

6. Taste the smoothie and adjust sweetness or thickness if necessary.

7. Pour the smoothie into a glass.

8. Garnish with a slice of pineapple or a kale leaf if desired.

9. Serve immediately and enjoy your nutritious Kale and Pineapple Smoothie!

Scrambled Eggs with Vegetables:

Ingredients:

- 3 large eggs
- 1/4 cup bell peppers, diced (assorted colors)
- 1/4 cup cherry tomatoes, halved
- 1/4 cup spinach, chopped
- 1/4 cup onion, finely chopped
- 1 clove garlic, minced
- 2 tablespoons milk
- 1 tablespoon olive oil or butter
- Salt and pepper to taste
- Fresh herbs (e.g., parsley or chives) for garnish (optional)

Instructions:

1. In a bowl, whisk together the eggs and milk until well combined. Season with salt and pepper.

2. Heat olive oil or butter in a non-stick skillet over medium heat.

3. Add chopped onions and minced garlic to the skillet. Sauté until softened and fragrant.

4. Add diced bell peppers to the skillet and cook until slightly tender.

5. Toss in the cherry tomatoes and chopped spinach. Cook until the spinach wilts and tomatoes soften.

6. Push the vegetables to one side of the skillet and pour the whisked eggs into the empty side.

7. Allow the eggs to set slightly around the edges before gently stirring, incorporating the vegetables.

8. Continue stirring occasionally until the eggs are fully cooked but still moist.

9. Remove the skillet from heat to prevent overcooking.

10. Garnish with fresh herbs if desired and serve the Scrambled Eggs with Vegetables immediately.

Chia Seed Pudding:

Ingredients:

- 1/4 cup chia seeds
- 1 cup milk (dairy or plant-based)
- 1-2 tablespoons honey or maple syrup (adjust to taste)
- 1/2 teaspoon vanilla extract
- Fresh fruits, nuts, or granola for topping (optional)

Instructions:

1. In a bowl, combine chia seeds, milk, honey or maple syrup, and vanilla extract.

2. Whisk the ingredients together until well combined. Ensure that the chia seeds are evenly distributed.

3. Let the mixture sit for about 5 minutes, then whisk again to prevent clumping.

4. Cover the bowl and refrigerate for at least 2 hours or overnight. Stir once or twice during the first hour to prevent chia seeds from settling at the bottom.

5. After refrigeration, the chia seeds will absorb the liquid and form a pudding-like consistency.

6. Give the pudding a good stir before serving to achieve a smooth texture.

7. Spoon the chia seed pudding into serving bowls or jars.

8. Top with fresh fruits, nuts, or granola for added texture and flavor.

9. Serve the Chia Seed Pudding chilled.

Turkey Sausage and Sweet Potato Hash:

Ingredients:

- 1 pound sweet potatoes, peeled and diced into small cubes
- 1/2 pound lean turkey sausage, crumbled
- 1 red bell pepper, diced
- 1 small onion, finely chopped
- 2 cloves garlic, minced
- 1 teaspoon smoked paprika
- 1/2 teaspoon ground cumin
- Salt and pepper to taste
- 2 tablespoons olive oil
- Fresh parsley for garnish (optional)
- Eggs (optional, for serving on top)

Instructions:

1. In a large skillet, heat olive oil over medium heat.

2. Add diced sweet potatoes to the skillet and cook for 5-7 minutes until they start to soften.

3. Add the crumbled turkey sausage to the skillet. Cook until the sausage is browned and cooked through.

4. Stir in the diced red bell pepper, chopped onion, and minced garlic. Sauté until the vegetables are tender.

5. Sprinkle smoked paprika, ground cumin, salt, and pepper over the mixture. Stir well to evenly coat everything with the spices.

6. Continue cooking for an additional 5-7 minutes until the sweet potatoes are fully cooked and slightly crispy.

7. Adjust the seasoning to taste, adding more salt or pepper if needed.

8. If desired, cook eggs separately and serve them on top of the hash.

9. Garnish with fresh parsley for a burst of flavor and color.

10. Serve the Turkey Sausage and Sweet Potato Hash warm and enjoy a hearty and delicious meal.

Almond Butter and Banana Smoothie:

Ingredients:

- 1 ripe banana, peeled and sliced
- 2 tablespoons almond butter
- 1 cup almond milk (or any preferred milk)
- 1/2 cup Greek yogurt
- 1 tablespoon honey or maple syrup (optional, depending on sweetness preference)
- 1/2 teaspoon vanilla extract
- Ice cubes (optional)

Instructions:

1. Place the sliced banana, almond butter, almond milk, Greek yogurt, honey or maple syrup (if using), and vanilla extract in a blender.

2. If you prefer a colder smoothie, add a handful of ice cubes to the blender.

3. Blend the ingredients on high speed until the mixture is smooth and creamy.

4. Taste the smoothie and adjust sweetness or thickness if necessary.

5. Pour the Almond Butter and Banana Smoothie into a glass.

6. Optionally, drizzle a little almond butter on top for extra flavor.

7. Serve immediately and enjoy this delicious and nutritious smoothie.

Frittata with Vegetables and Feta:

Ingredients:

- 6 large eggs
- 1/2 cup bell peppers, diced (assorted colors)
- 1/2 cup cherry tomatoes, halved

- 1/2 cup spinach, chopped
- 1/4 cup red onion, finely chopped
- 1/4 cup feta cheese, crumbled
- 2 tablespoons fresh herbs (e.g., parsley or chives), chopped
- 2 tablespoons olive oil
- Salt and pepper to taste

Instructions:

1. Preheat your oven to 375°F (190°C).
2. In a bowl, whisk the eggs until well beaten. Season with salt and pepper.
3. Heat olive oil in an oven-safe skillet over medium heat.
4. Add diced red onion to the skillet and sauté until softened.
5. Add bell peppers and cherry tomatoes to the skillet. Cook until the vegetables are slightly tender.
6. Toss in chopped spinach and cook until wilted.
7. Pour the beaten eggs over the vegetables in the skillet.
8. Allow the eggs to set around the edges. Lift the edges with a spatula to let the uncooked eggs flow underneath.
9. Sprinkle crumbled feta cheese evenly over the frittata.
10. Transfer the skillet to the preheated oven and bake for 12-15 minutes or until the frittata is set in the middle and slightly golden on top.
11. Carefully remove the skillet from the oven (use oven mitts as the handle will be hot).
12. Garnish with fresh herbs.
13. Allow the frittata to cool for a few minutes before slicing.
14. Serve the Vegetable and Feta Frittata warm, either as a main dish or a flavorful brunch option.

Grilled Chicken Salad:

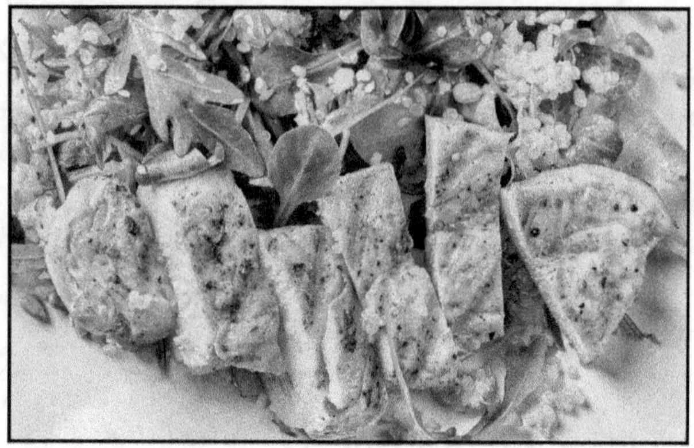

Ingredients:

For the Grilled Chicken:

- 2 boneless, skinless chicken breasts
- 2 tablespoons olive oil
- 1 teaspoon dried oregano
- 1 teaspoon garlic powder
- Salt and pepper to taste

For the Salad:

- Mixed salad greens (lettuce, spinach, arugula, etc.)
- Cherry tomatoes, halved
- Cucumber, sliced
- Red onion, thinly sliced
- Avocado, sliced
- Feta cheese, crumbled (optional)
- Kalamata olives (optional)

For the Dressing:

- 3 tablespoons extra-virgin olive oil
- 1 tablespoon balsamic vinegar
- 1 teaspoon Dijon mustard
- 1 clove garlic, minced
- Salt and pepper to taste

Instructions:

Grilled Chicken:

1. Preheat the grill or grill pan over medium-high heat.
2. In a bowl, mix olive oil, dried oregano, garlic powder, salt, and pepper.
3. Brush the chicken breasts with the prepared mixture on both sides.
4. Grill the chicken for about 6-8 minutes per side or until fully cooked (internal temperature of 165°F or 74°C).
5. Remove from the grill and let the chicken rest for a few minutes before slicing.

Salad:

6. In a large salad bowl, combine mixed greens, cherry tomatoes, cucumber, red onion, avocado, and any additional optional ingredients.

Dressing:

7. In a small bowl, whisk together olive oil, balsamic vinegar, Dijon mustard, minced garlic, salt, and pepper.

8. Drizzle the dressing over the salad and toss gently to combine.

Assembly:

9. Slice the grilled chicken and arrange it on top of the salad.

10. If desired, sprinkle crumbled feta cheese and Kalamata olives over the salad.

11. Serve the Grilled Chicken Salad immediately, offering any remaining dressing on the side.

Lentil Soup with Vegetables:

Ingredients:

- 1 cup dried green or brown lentils, rinsed and drained
- 1 onion, diced
- 2 carrots, diced
- 2 celery stalks, diced
- 3 cloves garlic, minced
- 1 can (14 oz) diced tomatoes
- 6 cups vegetable or chicken broth
- 1 teaspoon ground cumin
- 1 teaspoon ground coriander
- 1 teaspoon paprika
- 1/2 teaspoon turmeric (optional)
- Salt and pepper to taste
- 2 tablespoons olive oil
- Fresh lemon wedges for serving
- Fresh parsley for garnish (optional)

Instructions:

1. In a large pot, heat olive oil over medium heat.
2. Add diced onion, carrots, and celery. Sauté until the vegetables are softened.
3. Add minced garlic, cumin, coriander, paprika, and turmeric (if using). Stir well to coat the vegetables in the spices.
4. Pour in the rinsed lentils, diced tomatoes (with their juice), and vegetable or chicken broth.
5. Season with salt and pepper to taste. Bring the soup to a boil.
6. Reduce the heat to low, cover, and simmer for about 25-30 minutes or until the lentils are tender.
7. Taste and adjust the seasoning if needed.
8. Ladle the Lentil Soup into bowls.
9. Garnish with fresh parsley if desired and serve with lemon wedges on the side.
10. Enjoy this hearty and nutritious Lentil Soup with Vegetables!

Turkey and Avocado Wrap:

Ingredients:

- 1 large whole-grain or spinach tortilla
- 4 ounces cooked turkey breast, thinly sliced
- 1/2 avocado, sliced
- 1/4 cup cherry tomatoes, halved
- 1/4 cup cucumber, thinly sliced
- 2 tablespoons Greek yogurt or hummus
- 1 tablespoon Dijon mustard (optional)
- Fresh lettuce leaves
- Salt and pepper to taste

Instructions:

1. Lay the tortilla flat on a clean surface or plate.
2. In the center of the tortilla, spread a layer of Greek yogurt or hummus, leaving about an inch border around the edges.
3. Place the thinly sliced turkey evenly over the yogurt or hummus layer.
4. Arrange avocado slices, cherry tomatoes, and cucumber on top of the turkey.
5. If desired, add Dijon mustard for an extra kick.
6. Season with salt and pepper to taste.
7. Place fresh lettuce leaves over the ingredients.
8. Fold in the sides of the tortilla and then roll it up tightly from the bottom, creating a wrap.
9. Cut the wrap in half diagonally for easier handling, if preferred.
10. Serve immediately, or wrap in parchment paper for an on-the-go meal.

Quinoa Bowl with Black Beans and Salsa:

Ingredients:

For the Quinoa:

- 1 cup quinoa, rinsed and drained

- 2 cups water or vegetable broth
- 1/2 teaspoon salt

For the Black Beans:

- 1 can (15 oz) black beans, drained and rinsed
- 1 teaspoon ground cumin
- 1/2 teaspoon chili powder
- Salt and pepper to taste

For the Salsa:

- 1 cup cherry tomatoes, diced
- 1/2 red onion, finely chopped
- 1 jalapeño, seeded and finely chopped (optional for spice)
- 1/4 cup fresh cilantro, chopped
- 1 lime, juiced
- Salt and pepper to taste

Additional Toppings:

- Avocado slices
- Greek yogurt or sour cream
- Shredded cheese
- Lime wedges
- Fresh cilantro for garnish

Instructions:

Quinoa:

1. In a medium saucepan, combine quinoa, water or vegetable broth, and salt.
2. Bring to a boil, then reduce the heat to low, cover, and simmer for about 15-20 minutes or until the quinoa is cooked and the liquid is absorbed.
3. Fluff the quinoa with a fork.

Black Beans:

4. In a small saucepan, combine black beans, ground cumin, chili powder, salt, and pepper.

5. Cook over medium heat until the beans are heated through and the spices are well incorporated. Stir occasionally.

Salsa:

6. In a bowl, combine diced cherry tomatoes, chopped red onion, jalapeño (if using), cilantro, lime juice, salt, and pepper. Mix well.

Assembly:

7. Assemble your Quinoa Bowl by placing a portion of cooked quinoa in each bowl.

8. Top with seasoned black beans and a generous scoop of salsa.

9. Add avocado slices, a dollop of Greek yogurt or sour cream, and shredded cheese if desired.

10. Garnish with lime wedges and fresh cilantro.

11. Serve your Quinoa Bowl with Black Beans and Salsa immediately, allowing everyone to customize their toppings.

Tuna Salad Lettuce Wraps:

Ingredients:

For the Tuna Salad:

- 2 cans (5 oz each) tuna, drained
- 1/4 cup mayonnaise
- 1 tablespoon Dijon mustard
- 1 celery stalk, finely chopped
- 1/4 red onion, finely chopped
- 1 tablespoon fresh lemon juice
- Salt and pepper to taste

For the Lettuce Wraps:

- Large lettuce leaves (such as iceberg or butter lettuce)

Optional Toppings:

- Sliced cucumber
- Cherry tomatoes, halved

- Avocado slices
- Radish slices
- Fresh herbs (e.g., parsley or cilantro)

Instructions:

Tuna Salad:

1. In a bowl, combine drained tuna, mayonnaise, Dijon mustard, chopped celery, chopped red onion, and fresh lemon juice.
2. Mix until all the ingredients are well combined.
3. Season the tuna salad with salt and pepper to taste. Adjust the seasoning as needed.

Lettuce Wraps:

4. Wash and pat dry large lettuce leaves, ensuring they are intact for wrapping.

5. Spoon a portion of the tuna salad onto the center of each lettuce leaf.

Assembly:

6. Add your choice of optional toppings such as sliced cucumber, cherry tomatoes, avocado slices, radish slices, or fresh herbs.

7. Carefully fold or roll the lettuce leaves around the tuna salad and toppings, creating a wrap.
8. Secure the wraps with toothpicks if needed.
9. Arrange the Tuna Salad Lettuce Wraps on a serving platter.
10. Serve immediately, offering additional toppings or a wedge of lemon on the side.

Chicken and Vegetable Stir-Fry:

Ingredients:

For the Stir-Fry Sauce:

- 3 tablespoons soy sauce
- 2 tablespoons oyster sauce
- 1 tablespoon hoisin sauce
- 1 tablespoon rice vinegar

- 1 tablespoon honey
- 1 teaspoon sesame oil
- 1 teaspoon cornstarch (optional, for thickening)

For the Stir-Fry:

- 1 pound boneless, skinless chicken breasts, thinly sliced
- 2 tablespoons vegetable oil, divided
- 2 cups broccoli florets
- 1 red bell pepper, thinly sliced
- 1 carrot, julienned
- 1 cup snap peas, trimmed
- 3 green onions, sliced
- 3 cloves garlic, minced
- 1 tablespoon fresh ginger, grated
- Sesame seeds for garnish (optional)
- Cooked rice or noodles for serving

Instructions:

Stir-Fry Sauce:

1. In a bowl, whisk together soy sauce, oyster sauce, hoisin sauce, rice vinegar, honey, sesame oil, and cornstarch (if using). Set aside.

Chicken and Vegetable Stir-Fry:

2. Heat 1 tablespoon of vegetable oil in a large wok or skillet over medium-high heat.

3. Add sliced chicken to the pan and stir-fry until browned and cooked through. Remove the chicken from the pan and set aside.

4. In the same pan, add another tablespoon of oil.

5. Add minced garlic and grated ginger to the pan, stir-frying for about 30 seconds until fragrant.

6. Add broccoli, red bell pepper, julienned carrot, and snap peas to the pan. Stir-fry the vegetables for 3-5 minutes until they are crisp-tender.

7. Return the cooked chicken to the pan along with sliced green onions.

8. Pour the prepared stir-fry sauce over the chicken and vegetables.

9. Toss everything together until the chicken and vegetables are coated in the sauce. Cook for an additional 2-3 minutes until heated through.

10. Taste and adjust the seasoning if necessary.

11. Serve the Chicken and Vegetable Stir-Fry over cooked rice or noodles.

12. Garnish with sesame seeds if desired.

Spinach and Feta Stuffed Chicken Breast:

Ingredients:

- 4 boneless, skinless chicken breasts
- Salt and pepper to taste
- 1 tablespoon olive oil

For the Spinach and Feta Filling:

- 1 cup fresh spinach, chopped
- 1/2 cup feta cheese, crumbled
- 2 tablespoons cream cheese
- 2 cloves garlic, minced
- 1 tablespoon olive oil
- Salt and pepper to taste

For the Coating:

- 1/2 cup breadcrumbs
- 1/4 cup grated Parmesan cheese
- 1 teaspoon dried oregano
- 1 teaspoon paprika
- Olive oil spray (optional)

Instructions:

Prepare the Spinach and Feta Filling:

1. In a skillet, heat 1 tablespoon of olive oil over medium heat.

2. Add minced garlic and chopped spinach. Sauté until the spinach wilts.

3. Transfer the spinach and garlic to a bowl. Allow it to cool slightly.

4. Add feta cheese, cream cheese, salt, and pepper to the bowl. Mix well to combine.

Prepare the Chicken Breasts:

5. Preheat the oven to 375°F (190°C).

6. Using a sharp knife, make a horizontal slit along the side of each chicken breast to create a pocket.

7. Season the chicken breasts with salt and pepper.

8. Stuff each chicken breast with the spinach and feta filling, distributing it evenly among the pockets.

Coat and Cook the Chicken:

9. In a shallow bowl, combine breadcrumbs, Parmesan cheese, dried oregano, and paprika.

10. Roll each stuffed chicken breast in the breadcrumb mixture, ensuring an even coating.

11. Heat 1 tablespoon of olive oil in an oven-safe skillet over medium-high heat.

12. Sear the chicken breasts on each side until golden brown.

13. If desired, lightly spray the top of the chicken with olive oil.

14. Transfer the skillet to the preheated oven and bake for 20-25 minutes or until the chicken is cooked through.

15. Remove from the oven and let the Spinach and Feta Stuffed Chicken Breast rest for a few minutes before serving.

16. Serve the stuffed chicken breasts with your favorite side dishes.

Turkey Burger Lettuce Wraps:

Ingredients:

For the Turkey Patties:

- 1 pound ground turkey
- 1/4 cup breadcrumbs (gluten-free if needed)
- 1/4 cup grated Parmesan cheese

- 1/4 cup red onion, finely chopped
- 1 clove garlic, minced
- 1 teaspoon dried oregano
- 1 teaspoon Worcestershire sauce
- Salt and pepper to taste
- Olive oil for cooking

For Assembling Lettuce Wraps:

- Large lettuce leaves (such as iceberg or butter lettuce)
- Sliced tomatoes
- Red onion rings
- Avocado slices
- Mustard or your favorite condiments

Instructions:

Prepare Turkey Patties:

1. In a bowl, combine ground turkey, breadcrumbs, Parmesan cheese, chopped red onion, minced garlic, dried oregano, Worcestershire sauce, salt, and pepper.
2. Mix until all ingredients are well combined.
3. Divide the mixture into equal portions and shape them into burger patties.
4. Heat olive oil in a skillet over medium heat.
5. Cook the turkey patties for 4-5 minutes per side or until they are cooked through and have a golden-brown crust.

Assembling Turkey Burger Lettuce Wraps:

6. Wash and pat dry large lettuce leaves, ensuring they are intact for wrapping.
7. Place a turkey patty on each lettuce leaf.
8. Top with sliced tomatoes, red onion rings, and avocado slices.
9. Add your favorite condiments such as mustard or any other sauces.
10. Carefully fold or roll the lettuce leaves around the turkey patties and toppings, creating a wrap.
11. Secure the wraps with toothpicks if needed.

12. Serve the Turkey Burger Lettuce Wraps immediately.

Salmon with Quinoa and Asparagus:

Ingredients:

For the Salmon:

- 4 salmon fillets
- 2 tablespoons olive oil
- 2 cloves garlic, minced
- 1 teaspoon lemon zest
- 1 tablespoon lemon juice
- 1 teaspoon dried thyme (or fresh thyme)
- Salt and pepper to taste

For the Quinoa:

- 1 cup quinoa, rinsed
- 2 cups vegetable or chicken broth
- Salt to taste

For the Asparagus:

- 1 bunch asparagus, trimmed
- 1 tablespoon olive oil
- Salt and pepper to taste

For Garnish:

- Fresh parsley, chopped
- Lemon wedges

Instructions:

Prepare the Salmon:

1. Preheat the oven to 400°F (200°C).
2. In a small bowl, mix olive oil, minced garlic, lemon zest, lemon juice, dried thyme, salt, and pepper.
3. Place salmon fillets on a baking sheet lined with parchment paper.

4. Brush the salmon fillets with the prepared olive oil mixture.

5. Bake in the preheated oven for 12-15 minutes or until the salmon is cooked through and flakes easily with a fork.

Cook the Quinoa:

6. In a saucepan, combine quinoa and broth. Bring to a boil.

7. Reduce heat, cover, and simmer for 15-20 minutes or until the quinoa is cooked and the liquid is absorbed.

8. Fluff the quinoa with a fork and season with salt to taste.

Prepare the Asparagus:

9. Toss trimmed asparagus with olive oil, salt, and pepper.

10. Roast in the oven for about 10-12 minutes or until the asparagus is tender but still crisp.

Assemble the Dish:

11. Arrange a serving of cooked quinoa on each plate.

12. Top with a salmon fillet and a portion of roasted asparagus.

13. Garnish with chopped fresh parsley and serve with lemon wedges.

14. Enjoy this nutritious and flavorful Salmon with Quinoa and Asparagus!

Mediterranean Chickpea Salad:

Ingredients:

For the Salad:

- 2 cans (15 oz each) chickpeas, drained and rinsed
- 1 cucumber, diced
- 1 cup cherry tomatoes, halved
- 1/2 red onion, finely chopped
- 1/2 cup Kalamata olives, sliced
- 1/2 cup feta cheese, crumbled
- 1/4 cup fresh parsley, chopped

For the Dressing:

- 1/4 cup extra-virgin olive oil
- 2 tablespoons red wine vinegar
- 1 teaspoon Dijon mustard
- 1 clove garlic, minced
- 1 teaspoon dried oregano
- Salt and pepper to taste

Instructions:

Prepare the Salad:

1. In a large bowl, combine chickpeas, diced cucumber, halved cherry tomatoes, chopped red onion, sliced Kalamata olives, crumbled feta cheese, and chopped fresh parsley.

Make the Dressing:

2. In a small bowl or jar, whisk together olive oil, red wine vinegar, Dijon mustard, minced garlic, dried oregano, salt, and pepper.

Assemble the Salad:

3. Pour the dressing over the salad ingredients.

4. Toss everything together until the salad is well coated with the dressing.

5. Allow the Mediterranean Chickpea Salad to marinate for at least 15-20 minutes to enhance the flavors.

6. Taste and adjust the seasoning if necessary.

7. Serve the salad chilled.

CHAPTER 4: DINNER RECIPES

Baked Cod with Quinoa and Roasted Vegetables:

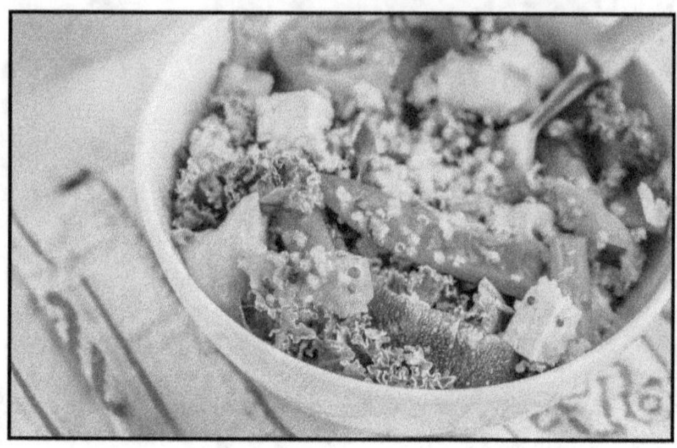

Ingredients:

- 4 cod fillets
- 1 cup quinoa, rinsed
- 2 cups mixed vegetables (e.g., bell peppers, zucchini, cherry tomatoes)
- 2 tablespoons olive oil
- 1 lemon, juiced
- 2 cloves garlic, minced
- 1 teaspoon dried oregano
- Salt and pepper to taste

Instructions:

1. Preheat the oven to 400°F (200°C).
2. Cook quinoa according to package instructions, using a 2:1 ratio of water to quinoa. Set aside.
3. In a bowl, mix olive oil, lemon juice, minced garlic, dried oregano, salt, and pepper to create a marinade.

4. Place cod fillets in a shallow dish and pour half of the marinade over them. Let it marinate for at least 15 minutes.

5. While the cod is marinating, chop the mixed vegetables into bite-sized pieces.

6. Toss the vegetables with the remaining marinade and spread them on a baking sheet.

7. Place the marinated cod fillets on the same baking sheet with the vegetables.

8. Bake in the preheated oven for about 15-20 minutes or until the cod is cooked through and flakes easily with a fork.

9. While the cod and vegetables are baking, fluff the cooked quinoa with a fork.

10. Serve the baked cod on a bed of quinoa with the roasted vegetables on the side. Garnish with fresh herbs if desired.

Beef Stir-Fry with Broccoli and Brown Rice:

Ingredients:

- 1 lb (450g) sirloin or flank steak, thinly sliced
- 3 cups broccoli florets
- 1 cup brown rice, cooked
- 3 tablespoons soy sauce
- 2 tablespoons oyster sauce
- 2 tablespoons hoisin sauce
- 1 tablespoon cornstarch
- 2 tablespoons vegetable oil
- 3 garlic cloves, minced
- 1 tablespoon ginger, minced
- 2 green onions, sliced (for garnish)
- Sesame seeds (optional, for garnish)

Instructions:

1. In a small bowl, mix soy sauce, oyster sauce, hoisin sauce, and cornstarch to create the marinade.

2. Place sliced beef in a bowl and pour half of the marinade over it. Allow it to marinate for at least 15-20 minutes.

3. Heat vegetable oil in a wok or large skillet over medium-high heat. Add minced garlic and ginger, and stir-fry for about 30 seconds.

4. Add marinated beef to the wok, stirring constantly until it's cooked through. Remove the beef from the wok and set it aside.

5. In the same wok, add a bit more oil if needed, then stir-fry broccoli until tender but still crisp.

6. Return the cooked beef to the wok, and add the remaining marinade. Stir to combine and cook for an additional 2-3 minutes.

7. Serve the beef and broccoli stir-fry over cooked brown rice.

8. Garnish with sliced green onions and sesame seeds if desired.

Grilled Shrimp with Sweet Potato Wedges:

Ingredients:

- 1 lb (450g) large shrimp, peeled and deveined
- 2 large sweet potatoes, cut into wedges
- 2 tablespoons olive oil
- 1 teaspoon smoked paprika
- 1 teaspoon garlic powder
- 1 teaspoon dried oregano
- Salt and black pepper to taste
- Wooden skewers (pre-soaked in water if using)

Instructions:

1. Preheat your grill to medium-high heat.

2. In a bowl, toss the shrimp with olive oil, smoked paprika, garlic powder, dried oregano, salt, and black pepper. Ensure the shrimp are well-coated and set aside to marinate for at least 15 minutes.

3. Meanwhile, preheat your oven to 400°F (200°C).

4. Toss sweet potato wedges with olive oil, salt, and pepper. Place them on a baking sheet in a single layer.

5. Roast sweet potato wedges in the preheated oven for 20-25 minutes or until they are golden and tender.

6. Thread marinated shrimp onto skewers, leaving a small space between each shrimp.

7. Grill the shrimp skewers for 2-3 minutes per side or until they are opaque and cooked through.

8. Serve the grilled shrimp alongside the roasted sweet potato wedges.

Chicken and Vegetable Skewers with Quinoa:

Ingredients:

- 1 lb (450g) boneless, skinless chicken breasts, cut into chunks
- 2 bell peppers (any color), cut into chunks
- 1 zucchini, sliced into rounds
- 1 red onion, cut into chunks
- 1 cup quinoa
- 2 cups chicken broth or water
- 3 tablespoons olive oil
- 2 tablespoons lemon juice
- 2 teaspoons dried oregano
- 1 teaspoon garlic powder
- Salt and black pepper to taste
- Wooden skewers (pre-soaked in water if using)

Instructions:

1. In a bowl, whisk together olive oil, lemon juice, dried oregano, garlic powder, salt, and black pepper to create the marinade.

2. Thread chicken chunks, bell peppers, zucchini slices, and red onion chunks onto the skewers, alternating between them.

3. Brush the skewers with the prepared marinade, ensuring all sides are coated. Allow them to marinate for at least 15 minutes.

4. While the skewers marinate, rinse quinoa under cold water. In a saucepan, combine quinoa and chicken broth (or water). Bring to a boil, then reduce heat, cover, and simmer for 15 minutes or until quinoa is cooked and liquid is absorbed.

5. Preheat your grill or grill pan to medium-high heat.

6. Grill the skewers for 4-5 minutes per side or until the chicken is cooked through and the vegetables are slightly charred.

7. Serve the chicken and vegetable skewers over a bed of cooked quinoa.

Quinoa Bowl with Mixed Beans and Salsa:

Ingredients:

- 1 cup quinoa, rinsed
- 2 cups water or vegetable broth
- 1 can (15 oz) mixed beans (such as black beans, kidney beans, or pinto beans), drained and rinsed
- 1 cup corn kernels (fresh or frozen)
- 1 cup cherry tomatoes, halved
- 1/2 red onion, finely diced
- 1 jalapeño, finely diced (seeds removed for less heat)
- 1/4 cup fresh cilantro, chopped
- Juice of 2 limes
- 2 tablespoons olive oil
- 1 teaspoon ground cumin
- Salt and black pepper to taste
- Avocado slices for garnish (optional)

Instructions:

1. In a saucepan, combine quinoa and water (or vegetable broth). Bring to a boil, then reduce heat, cover, and simmer for 15 minutes or until quinoa is cooked and liquid is absorbed.

2. In a large bowl, combine mixed beans, corn, cherry tomatoes, red onion, jalapeño, and cilantro.

3. In a small bowl, whisk together lime juice, olive oil, ground cumin, salt, and black pepper to create the dressing.

4. Fluff the cooked quinoa with a fork and add it to the bowl with the mixed beans and vegetables.

5. Pour the dressing over the quinoa and bean mixture. Toss everything together until well combined.

6. Taste and adjust seasoning if necessary.

7. Serve the quinoa bowl with mixed beans and salsa in individual bowls, garnishing with avocado slices if desired.

Turkey Meatballs with Zucchini Noodles:

Ingredients:
For Turkey Meatballs:
- 1 lb (450g) ground turkey
- 1/2 cup breadcrumbs
- 1/4 cup grated Parmesan cheese
- 1 large egg
- 2 cloves garlic, minced
- 1 teaspoon dried oregano
- 1 teaspoon dried basil
- Salt and black pepper to taste
- 2 tablespoons olive oil (for baking)

For Zucchini Noodles:
- 4 medium-sized zucchinis, spiralized
- 2 tablespoons olive oil
- Salt and black pepper to taste

For Tomato Sauce:

- 1 can (14 oz) crushed tomatoes
- 2 cloves garlic, minced
- 1 teaspoon dried Italian herbs (basil, oregano, thyme)
- Salt and black pepper to taste

Instructions:

1. Turkey Meatballs:
    1. Preheat the oven to 375°F (190°C).
    2. In a bowl, combine ground turkey, breadcrumbs, Parmesan cheese, egg, minced garlic, dried oregano, dried basil, salt, and black pepper. Mix until well combined.
    3. Form the mixture into meatballs, about 1 to 1.5 inches in diameter.
    4. Place the meatballs on a baking sheet lined with parchment paper, drizzle with olive oil, and bake for 20-25 minutes or until cooked through and golden brown.
2. Zucchini Noodles:
    1. Spiralize the zucchinis into noodles.
    2. Heat olive oil in a large pan over medium heat. Add the zucchini noodles, season with salt and black pepper, and sauté for 2-3 minutes until they are just tender but still have a slight crunch.
3. Tomato Sauce:
    1. In a saucepan, combine crushed tomatoes, minced garlic, Italian herbs, salt, and black pepper. Simmer over low heat for about 10-15 minutes, allowing the flavors to meld.
4. Assembling:
    1. Place a portion of zucchini noodles on a plate, top with turkey meatballs, and drizzle with tomato sauce.
    2. Garnish with additional Parmesan cheese and fresh herbs if desired.

Salmon with Steamed Broccoli and Quinoa:

Ingredients:

- 4 salmon fillets
- 1 cup quinoa, rinsed
- 2 cups water or vegetable broth
- 1 lb (450g) broccoli florets
- 2 tablespoons olive oil
- 2 cloves garlic, minced
- Juice of 1 lemon
- Salt and black pepper to taste

- Fresh dill or parsley for garnish

Instructions:

1. Quinoa:
    1. In a saucepan, combine quinoa and water (or vegetable broth). Bring to a boil, then reduce heat, cover, and simmer for 15 minutes or until quinoa is cooked and liquid is absorbed.
2. Salmon:
    1. Preheat the oven to 400°F (200°C).
    2. Place salmon fillets on a baking sheet lined with parchment paper. Drizzle with olive oil and lemon juice.
    3. Season the salmon with minced garlic, salt, and black pepper.
    4. Bake in the preheated oven for 12-15 minutes or until the salmon is cooked through and flakes easily with a fork.
3. Broccoli:
    1. Steam the broccoli florets until they are tender but still vibrant, about 5-7 minutes.
4. Assembling:
    1. Place a serving of cooked quinoa on each plate.
    2. Top with a portion of steamed broccoli and a baked salmon fillet.
    3. Garnish with fresh dill or parsley.
    4. Serve with an extra squeeze of lemon if desired.

Chicken and Broccoli Stir-Fry with Cauliflower Rice:

Ingredients:

For Chicken and Broccoli Stir-Fry:
- 1 lb (450g) boneless, skinless chicken breasts, thinly sliced
- 3 cups broccoli florets
- 3 tablespoons soy sauce
- 1 tablespoon oyster sauce
- 1 tablespoon hoisin sauce
- 1 tablespoon cornstarch
- 2 tablespoons vegetable oil
- 3 cloves garlic, minced
- 1 tablespoon ginger, minced
- 2 green onions, sliced (for garnish)
- Sesame seeds (optional, for garnish)

For Cauliflower Rice:

- 1 large cauliflower, grated or processed into rice-like texture
- 2 tablespoons vegetable oil
- Salt and black pepper to taste

Instructions:

1. Chicken and Broccoli Stir-Fry:
    1. In a small bowl, mix soy sauce, oyster sauce, hoisin sauce, and cornstarch to create the sauce.
    2. Place sliced chicken in a bowl and pour half of the sauce over it. Allow it to marinate for at least 15-20 minutes.
    3. Heat vegetable oil in a wok or large skillet over medium-high heat. Add minced garlic and ginger, and stir-fry for about 30 seconds.
    4. Add the marinated chicken to the wok, stirring constantly until it's cooked through. Remove the chicken from the wok and set it aside.
    5. In the same wok, add a bit more oil if needed, then stir-fry broccoli until tender but still crisp.
    6. Return the cooked chicken to the wok, and add the remaining sauce. Stir to combine and cook for an additional 2-3 minutes.
    7. Garnish with sliced green onions and sesame seeds if desired.
2. Cauliflower Rice:
    1. In a separate pan, heat vegetable oil over medium heat.
    2. Add grated or processed cauliflower to the pan and sauté for 5-7 minutes until it's tender but not mushy.
    3. Season with salt and black pepper to taste.
3. Assembling:
    1. Serve the Chicken and Broccoli Stir-Fry over a bed of Cauliflower Rice.
    2. Garnish with additional green onions and sesame seeds if desired.

Baked Chicken Thighs with Sweet Potatoes and Brussels Sprouts:

Ingredients:

- 4 bone-in, skin-on chicken thighs
- 2 large sweet potatoes, peeled and cubed
- 1 lb (450g) Brussels sprouts, trimmed and halved
- 3 tablespoons olive oil
- 2 tablespoons balsamic vinegar
- 2 cloves garlic, minced

- 1 teaspoon dried thyme
- 1 teaspoon paprika
- Salt and black pepper to taste
- Fresh parsley for garnish

Instructions:

1. Preheat the oven to 425°F (220°C).
2. In a large bowl, combine sweet potato cubes and halved Brussels sprouts. Drizzle with 2 tablespoons of olive oil, balsamic vinegar, minced garlic, dried thyme, paprika, salt, and black pepper. Toss until the vegetables are well coated.
3. Season the chicken thighs with salt and pepper.
4. Heat the remaining 1 tablespoon of olive oil in an oven-safe skillet over medium-high heat. Add chicken thighs, skin side down, and sear for 3-4 minutes until the skin is golden brown.
5. Flip the chicken thighs and place them skin side up in the skillet, surrounded by the sweet potatoes and Brussels sprouts.
6. Transfer the skillet to the preheated oven and bake for 25-30 minutes or until the chicken is cooked through and the vegetables are tender.
7. Garnish with fresh parsley before serving.
8. Serve the baked chicken thighs with sweet potatoes and Brussels sprouts on a platter.

Shrimp and Vegetable Stir-Fry with Brown Rice:

Ingredients:

- 1 lb (450g) large shrimp, peeled and deveined
- 2 cups broccoli florets
- 1 bell pepper, thinly sliced
- 1 carrot, julienned
- 1 cup snap peas, trimmed
- 3 tablespoons soy sauce

- 2 tablespoons oyster sauce
- 1 tablespoon hoisin sauce
- 1 tablespoon cornstarch
- 2 tablespoons vegetable oil
- 3 cloves garlic, minced
- 1 tablespoon ginger, minced
- 4 cups cooked brown rice
- Green onions, sliced (for garnish)
- Sesame seeds (optional, for garnish)

Instructions:

1. In a small bowl, whisk together soy sauce, oyster sauce, hoisin sauce, and cornstarch to create the sauce.
2. Heat 1 tablespoon of vegetable oil in a wok or large skillet over medium-high heat. Add minced garlic and ginger, and stir-fry for about 30 seconds.
3. Add shrimp to the wok and cook until they turn pink, about 2-3 minutes. Remove the shrimp from the wok and set aside.
4. Heat the remaining tablespoon of oil in the wok. Add broccoli, bell pepper, carrot, and snap peas. Stir-fry the vegetables for 3-4 minutes until they are tender-crisp.
5. Return the cooked shrimp to the wok and pour the sauce over the shrimp and vegetables. Stir to combine and cook for an additional 2-3 minutes.
6. Serve the shrimp and vegetable stir-fry over cooked brown rice.

Turkey Chili with Mixed Vegetables:

Ingredients:

- 1 lb (450g) ground turkey
- 1 onion, finely diced
- 2 bell peppers (any color), diced
- 2 carrots, peeled and diced
- 2 celery stalks, diced

- 3 cloves garlic, minced
- 1 can (14 oz) diced tomatoes
- 1 can (15 oz) kidney beans, drained and rinsed
- 1 can (15 oz) black beans, drained and rinsed
- 1 cup corn kernels (fresh or frozen)
- 3 cups chicken or vegetable broth
- 2 tablespoons tomato paste
- 2 teaspoons ground cumin
- 1 tablespoon chili powder
- 1 teaspoon paprika
- 1/2 teaspoon oregano
- Salt and black pepper to taste
- Olive oil for cooking
- Optional toppings: shredded cheese, sour cream, chopped green onions, cilantro

Instructions:

1. In a large pot, heat olive oil over medium heat. Add diced onion, bell peppers, carrots, and celery. Sauté until the vegetables are softened, about 5-7 minutes.
2. Add minced garlic and ground turkey to the pot. Cook until the turkey is browned and cooked through.
3. Stir in tomato paste, ground cumin, chili powder, paprika, oregano, salt, and black pepper. Cook for an additional 2 minutes to enhance flavors.
4. Pour in diced tomatoes, kidney beans, black beans, corn, and chicken or vegetable broth. Bring the chili to a simmer and let it cook for 20-25 minutes, allowing the flavors to meld.
5. Adjust seasoning to taste and add more broth if needed for desired consistency.
6. Serve the turkey chili hot, topped with shredded cheese, sour cream, chopped green onions, or cilantro if desired.

CHAPTER 5: SNACK IDEAS FOR BLOOD TYPE O POSITIVE

Apple Slices with Almond Butter:

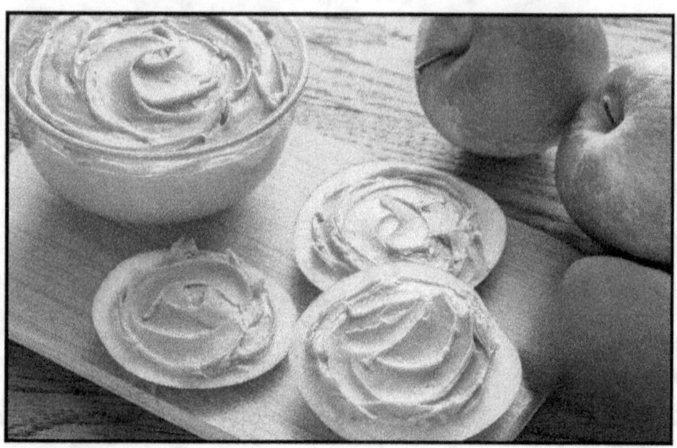

Ingredients:

- 2 medium-sized apples (any variety), cored and sliced
- 1/4 cup almond butter
- 1 tablespoon honey (optional)
- 1 teaspoon cinnamon (optional)
- Squeeze of lemon juice (to prevent browning)

Instructions:

1. Core and slice the apples into thin wedges.
2. Place the apple slices in a bowl and drizzle with a little lemon juice, tossing to coat. This helps prevent the apples from browning.
3. In a small microwave-safe bowl, warm the almond butter for about 15-20 seconds until it becomes slightly more fluid.
4. Arrange the apple slices on a plate or serving platter.
5. Drizzle almond butter over the apple slices or, if you prefer, dip each slice into the almond butter.

6. Optional: Drizzle honey over the almond butter for added sweetness and sprinkle with cinnamon.

7. Serve immediately and enjoy your delicious and healthy snack of Apple Slices with Almond Butter!

Carrot Sticks with Hummus:

Ingredients:

- 4 large carrots, peeled and cut into sticks
- 1 cup hummus (store-bought or homemade)
- Fresh parsley or paprika for garnish (optional)

Instructions:

1. Peel the carrots and cut them into sticks, ensuring they are of a size suitable for dipping.
2. Place the carrot sticks on a serving plate.
3. In a bowl or small serving dish, scoop out the hummus.
4. If desired, garnish the hummus with a sprinkle of fresh parsley or a dash of paprika for added flavor and visual appeal.
5. Arrange the carrot sticks around the hummus bowl.
6. Serve immediately and enjoy this healthy and satisfying snack of Carrot Sticks with Hummus!

Mixed Nuts:

Ingredients:

- 1 cup almonds
- 1 cup walnuts
- 1 cup cashews
- 1 cup pecans
- 1 cup mixed nuts of your choice (such as hazelnuts, pistachios, or macadamia nuts)

- 1 tablespoon melted butter or olive oil
- 1 teaspoon sea salt
- 1/2 teaspoon black pepper
- 1/2 teaspoon garlic powder (optional)
- 1/2 teaspoon paprika (optional)
- 1/4 teaspoon cayenne pepper (optional)

Instructions:

1. Preheat the oven to 350°F (175°C).
2. In a large mixing bowl, combine all the nuts.
3. In a small bowl, mix the melted butter or olive oil with sea salt, black pepper, and any optional seasonings you prefer, such as garlic powder, paprika, or cayenne pepper.
4. Pour the seasoned mixture over the nuts and toss until the nuts are evenly coated.
5. Spread the nuts in a single layer on a baking sheet lined with parchment paper.
6. Roast in the preheated oven for 10-15 minutes, stirring occasionally, until the nuts are golden and fragrant.
7. Remove from the oven and let the mixed nuts cool completely.
8. Once cooled, transfer the mixed nuts to an airtight container for storage.
9. Enjoy your homemade Mixed Nuts as a tasty and nutritious snack!

Greek Yogurt with Berries:

Ingredients:

- 1 cup Greek yogurt (plain or vanilla-flavored)
- 1/2 cup fresh berries (such as strawberries, blueberries, raspberries, or blackberries)
- 1 tablespoon honey or maple syrup (optional)
- 1/4 cup granola (optional)
- Fresh mint leaves for garnish (optional)

Instructions:

1. In a bowl, scoop out the Greek yogurt.

2. Wash and prepare the berries, cutting larger berries into bite-sized pieces if necessary.

3. Arrange the fresh berries on top of the Greek yogurt.

4. If you desire a touch of sweetness, drizzle honey or maple syrup over the berries.

5. Optionally, sprinkle granola over the yogurt and berries for added texture.

6. Garnish with fresh mint leaves for a burst of freshness.

7. Serve immediately and enjoy your delightful and nutritious Greek Yogurt with Berries!

Rice Cakes with Almond Butter:

Ingredients:

- 4 rice cakes
- 1/2 cup almond butter
- 1-2 tablespoons honey (optional)
- Sliced banana or berries for topping (optional)
- Chia seeds or crushed nuts for garnish (optional)

Instructions:

1. Spread a generous layer of almond butter evenly onto each rice cake.

2. Drizzle honey over the almond butter for added sweetness if desired.

3. Optional: Top with sliced banana, berries, chia seeds, or crushed nuts for extra flavor and texture.

4. Arrange the prepared rice cakes on a serving plate.

5. Serve immediately and enjoy your quick and satisfying snack of Rice Cakes with Almond Butter!

Cheese and Cherry Tomatoes:

Ingredients:

- 1 cup cherry tomatoes

- 1 cup bite-sized cheese cubes (cheddar, mozzarella, or your favorite cheese)
- Fresh basil leaves for garnish (optional)
- Balsamic glaze for drizzling (optional)
- Toothpicks or small skewers

Instructions:

1. Wash the cherry tomatoes and pat them dry.
2. Arrange a cherry tomato and a cheese cube on each toothpick or skewer. Repeat for the desired number of servings.
3. Optional: Garnish with fresh basil leaves for an extra burst of flavor.
4. If desired, drizzle balsamic glaze over the cheese and cherry tomato skewers.
5. Arrange the skewers on a serving platter.
6. Serve immediately, and enjoy this simple and delightful Cheese and Cherry Tomatoes snack!

Cottage Cheese with Pineapple Chunks:

Ingredients:

- 1 cup cottage cheese
- 1/2 cup fresh pineapple chunks
- 1 tablespoon honey (optional)
- Mint leaves for garnish (optional)

Instructions:

1. In a bowl, spoon out the cottage cheese.
2. Add fresh pineapple chunks to the cottage cheese.
3. If you prefer added sweetness, drizzle honey over the cottage cheese and pineapple.
4. Optional: Garnish with mint leaves for a touch of freshness.
5. Mix gently to combine the cottage cheese and pineapple.
6. Serve immediately and enjoy your light and refreshing Cottage Cheese with Pineapple Chunks!

Celery Sticks with Peanut Butter:

Ingredients:

- 4 celery stalks, washed and trimmed
- 1/2 cup peanut butter (smooth or crunchy)
- Raisins or chopped nuts for topping (optional)

Instructions:

1. Cut the celery stalks into manageable sticks, about 4-5 inches in length.
2. Spread peanut butter along the inner groove of each celery stick.
3. Optionally, top the peanut butter with raisins or chopped nuts for added texture and flavor.
4. Arrange the celery sticks on a serving plate.
5. Serve immediately and enjoy this classic and nutritious snack of Celery Sticks with Peanut Butter!

Hard-Boiled Eggs:

Ingredients:

- Eggs (as many as desired)

Instructions:

1. Place the eggs in a single layer in a saucepan or pot. You can cook as few or as many eggs as you like, depending on your needs.
2. Add enough water to the pot to cover the eggs by about an inch.
3. Place the pot on the stove over medium-high heat and bring the water to a boil.
4. Once the water is boiling, reduce the heat to low and let the eggs simmer for about 9-12 minutes, depending on your desired yolk consistency. Longer for fully set yolks, shorter for softer yolks.
5. While the eggs are simmering, prepare a bowl of ice water.
6. When the eggs are done, use a slotted spoon to transfer them to the bowl of ice water. Let them sit for a few minutes to cool and make peeling easier.

7. Once cooled, gently tap the eggs on a hard surface, roll them to loosen the shell, and peel under running water if needed.

8. Your hard-boiled eggs are ready to be enjoyed as a snack, sliced onto salads, or as a protein-packed addition to your meals.

Yogurt with Sliced Kiwi:

Ingredients:

- 1 cup plain or vanilla-flavored yogurt
- 2 ripe kiwis, peeled and sliced
- 1 tablespoon honey (optional)
- Granola or chopped nuts for topping (optional)

Instructions:

1. In a bowl, scoop out the desired amount of yogurt.
2. Peel and slice the ripe kiwis.
3. Arrange the kiwi slices on top of the yogurt.
4. If you prefer added sweetness, drizzle honey over the yogurt and kiwi.
5. Optionally, sprinkle granola or chopped nuts on top for added texture.
6. Serve immediately and enjoy your delicious and refreshing Yogurt with Sliced Kiwi!

Cherry Tomatoes with Mozzarella:

Ingredients:

- 1 cup cherry tomatoes, washed
- 1 cup fresh mozzarella balls (bocconcini)
- Fresh basil leaves
- Extra virgin olive oil
- Balsamic glaze (optional)
- Salt and black pepper to taste

Instructions:

1. On toothpicks or small skewers, thread one cherry tomato, followed by a mozzarella ball, and then a fresh basil leaf. Repeat for desired servings.

2. Arrange the tomato and mozzarella skewers on a serving plate.

3. Drizzle extra virgin olive oil over the skewers.

4. Optionally, if you desire a touch of sweetness, drizzle balsamic glaze over the tomato and mozzarella skewers.

5. Sprinkle with salt and black pepper to taste.

6. Serve immediately and enjoy this simple and flavorful appetizer of Cherry Tomatoes with Mozzarella!

CHAPTER 6: DESSERTS TAILORED FOR BLOOD TYPE O POSITIVE

Dark Chocolate Covered Berries:

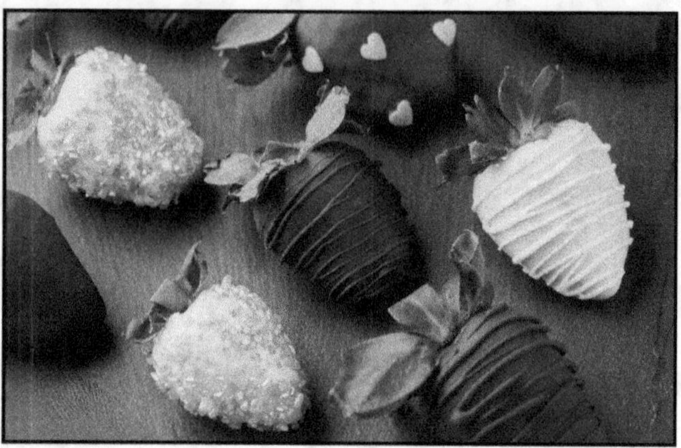

Ingredients:

- 1 cup dark chocolate chips or chopped dark chocolate
- 1 cup fresh berries (strawberries, blueberries, raspberries, or a mix)
- Optional: White chocolate for drizzling
- Optional: Chopped nuts or shredded coconut for coating

Instructions:

1. Wash and thoroughly dry the berries to ensure the chocolate adheres well.

2. In a heatproof bowl, melt the dark chocolate using a microwave or a double boiler. Stir frequently until smooth.

3. Holding each berry by the stem or using toothpicks, dip them into the melted dark chocolate, coating them evenly.

4. Allow any excess chocolate to drip off, then place the chocolate-covered berries on a parchment paper-lined tray.

5. If desired, drizzle melted white chocolate over the dark chocolate-covered berries for a decorative touch.

6. Optional: While the chocolate is still wet, roll the berries in chopped nuts or shredded coconut for added texture.

7. Allow the chocolate-covered berries to cool and set. You can place them in the refrigerator for faster setting.

8. Once the chocolate is completely set, transfer the dark chocolate-covered berries to a serving plate.

9. Serve and enjoy your delightful Dark Chocolate Covered Berries!

Almond Flour Banana Bread:

Ingredients:

- 3 ripe bananas, mashed
- 3 large eggs
- 1/4 cup coconut oil, melted (or melted butter)
- 1 teaspoon vanilla extract
- 2 cups almond flour
- 1/2 teaspoon baking soda
- 1/4 teaspoon salt
- 1 teaspoon ground cinnamon (optional)
- 1/2 cup chopped nuts or chocolate chips (optional)

Instructions:

1. Preheat your oven to 350°F (175°C). Grease a loaf pan or line it with parchment paper.

2. In a large bowl, mash the ripe bananas with a fork or potato masher.

3. Add the eggs, melted coconut oil (or butter), and vanilla extract to the mashed bananas. Mix well.

4. In a separate bowl, whisk together almond flour, baking soda, salt, and cinnamon if using.

5. Gradually add the dry ingredients to the wet ingredients, mixing until well combined.

6. If desired, fold in chopped nuts or chocolate chips into the batter.

7. Pour the batter into the prepared loaf pan, spreading it evenly.

8. Bake in the preheated oven for 45-55 minutes or until a toothpick inserted into the center comes out clean.

9. Allow the almond flour banana bread to cool in the pan for 10-15 minutes, then transfer it to a wire rack to cool completely.

10. Once cooled, slice and serve. Enjoy your delicious Almond Flour Banana Bread

Coconut Milk Chia Seed Pudding:

Ingredients:

- 1/4 cup chia seeds
- 1 cup coconut milk (full-fat for creamier texture)
- 1-2 tablespoons maple syrup or honey (adjust to taste)
- 1/2 teaspoon vanilla extract
- Optional toppings: Fresh berries, sliced fruits, shredded coconut, or nuts

Instructions:

1. In a bowl, combine chia seeds, coconut milk, maple syrup or honey, and vanilla extract.

2. Whisk the ingredients thoroughly to ensure the chia seeds are well distributed and don't clump together.

3. Cover the bowl and refrigerate for at least 3 hours or overnight to allow the chia seeds to absorb the liquid and create a pudding-like consistency.

4. After the initial refrigeration, give the mixture a good stir to break up any clumps. If it's too thick, you can add a little more coconut milk.

5. Taste and adjust sweetness if needed by adding more maple syrup or honey.

6. Serve the coconut milk chia seed pudding in individual jars or bowls.

7. Top with fresh berries, sliced fruits, shredded coconut, or nuts for added flavor and texture.

8. Enjoy your Coconut Milk Chia Seed Pudding as a healthy and satisfying breakfast or dessert!

Pumpkin Spice Baked Apples:

Ingredients:

- 4 medium-sized baking apples (such as Granny Smith or Honeycrisp)
- 1/2 cup chopped nuts (walnuts or pecans), optional
- 1/4 cup dried cranberries or raisins, optional
- 1/4 cup brown sugar or coconut sugar
- 2 tablespoons unsalted butter, melted
- 1 teaspoon ground cinnamon
- 1/2 teaspoon ground nutmeg
- 1/4 teaspoon ground cloves
- 1/4 teaspoon ground ginger
- 1/4 cup pure maple syrup
- Vanilla ice cream or whipped cream for serving, optional

Instructions:

1. Preheat your oven to 375°F (190°C).
2. Wash and core the apples, leaving the bottoms intact to create a well for the filling.
3. In a bowl, mix together chopped nuts, dried cranberries or raisins (if using), brown sugar, melted butter, ground cinnamon, ground nutmeg, ground cloves, and ground ginger.
4. Stuff each cored apple with the nut and spice mixture, pressing it down gently.
5. Place the stuffed apples in a baking dish.
6. Drizzle pure maple syrup over each apple, ensuring it gets into the filling.
7. Cover the baking dish with foil and bake in the preheated oven for 25-30 minutes or until the apples are tender.

8. Remove the foil and bake for an additional 5-10 minutes to allow the tops to brown slightly.

9. Serve the Pumpkin Spice Baked Apples warm, optionally topped with vanilla ice cream or whipped cream.

Avocado Chocolate Mousse:

Ingredients:

- 2 ripe avocados
- 1/4 cup cocoa powder
- 1/4 cup maple syrup or honey
- 1/4 cup milk (dairy or plant-based)
- 1 teaspoon vanilla extract
- A pinch of salt
- Optional toppings: Fresh berries, sliced banana, chopped nuts, or whipped cream

Instructions:

1. Cut the avocados in half, remove the pits, and scoop the flesh into a blender or food processor.

2. Add cocoa powder, maple syrup or honey, milk, vanilla extract, and a pinch of salt to the blender.

3. Blend the ingredients until smooth and creamy, scraping down the sides as needed to ensure everything is well combined.

4. Taste the chocolate mousse and adjust sweetness or cocoa powder if needed.

5. Refrigerate the avocado chocolate mousse for at least 1-2 hours to allow it to chill and firm up.

6. Once chilled, spoon the mousse into serving bowls or glasses.

7. Top with fresh berries, sliced banana, chopped nuts, or a dollop of whipped cream if desired.

8. Serve and enjoy your delicious and healthier Avocado Chocolate Mousse!

Mixed Berry Sorbet:

Ingredients:

- 3 cups mixed berries (strawberries, blueberries, raspberries, blackberries)
- 1/2 cup granulated sugar
- 1 tablespoon fresh lemon juice
- 1 cup water

Instructions:

1. Wash the mixed berries thoroughly and remove any stems.
2. In a saucepan, combine water and sugar. Heat over medium heat, stirring until the sugar is completely dissolved. Allow the sugar syrup to cool.
3. Place the mixed berries and fresh lemon juice in a blender or food processor.
4. Pour the cooled sugar syrup into the blender with the berries.
5. Blend until the mixture is smooth and well combined.
6. Strain the berry mixture through a fine-mesh sieve to remove seeds and pulp, if desired, for a smoother sorbet.
7. Transfer the strained mixture to an ice cream maker and churn according to the manufacturer's instructions until it reaches a sorbet-like consistency.
8. If you don't have an ice cream maker, pour the mixture into a shallow dish and place it in the freezer. Every 30 minutes, stir the mixture with a fork to break up ice crystals, repeating until the sorbet is frozen.
9. Once the sorbet reaches your desired consistency, transfer it to an airtight container and freeze for an additional 2-3 hours.
10. Scoop and serve the Mixed Berry Sorbet in bowls or cones.
11. Enjoy the refreshing and fruity taste of your homemade Mixed Berry Sorbet!

Walnut and Date Energy Bites:

Ingredients:

- 1 cup walnuts
- 1 cup pitted dates

- 1/4 cup unsweetened shredded coconut
- 1 tablespoon chia seeds
- 1/2 teaspoon vanilla extract
- A pinch of salt (optional)
- Additional shredded coconut for rolling (optional)

Instructions:

1. In a food processor, combine walnuts, pitted dates, shredded coconut, chia seeds, vanilla extract, and a pinch of salt.
2. Process the ingredients until the mixture becomes a sticky, uniform dough. If the mixture is too dry, you can add a few more dates.
3. Scoop out about a tablespoon of the mixture and roll it between your hands to form a compact ball.
4. If desired, roll the energy bites in additional shredded coconut for extra flavor and texture.
5. Repeat the process until all the mixture is used.
6. Place the Walnut and Date Energy Bites on a plate or tray and refrigerate for at least 30 minutes to firm up.
7. Once firm, transfer the energy bites to an airtight container and store them in the refrigerator for longer shelf life.
8. Enjoy these nutritious and delicious Walnut and Date Energy Bites as a quick and energizing snack!

Baked Pears with Cinnamon:

Ingredients:

- 4 ripe but firm pears
- 2 tablespoons unsalted butter, melted
- 2 tablespoons honey or maple syrup
- 1 teaspoon ground cinnamon
- Optional toppings: Greek yogurt, vanilla ice cream, or chopped nuts

Instructions:

1. Preheat your oven to 375°F (190°C).
2. Wash and halve the pears. Core each half, creating a small well for the filling.
3. In a small bowl, mix melted butter, honey or maple syrup, and ground cinnamon.
4. Place the pear halves in a baking dish, cut side up.
5. Brush the melted butter mixture over the top of each pear half, ensuring they are well coated.
6. Bake in the preheated oven for 25-30 minutes or until the pears are tender and the edges start to caramelize.
7. Optionally, spoon any juices from the baking dish over the pears during baking to enhance the flavors.
8. Remove from the oven and let the baked pears cool slightly.
9. Serve the Baked Pears with Cinnamon warm, optionally topped with a dollop of Greek yogurt, a scoop of vanilla ice cream, or a sprinkle of chopped nuts.

Coconut Yogurt Parfait:

Ingredients:

- 1 cup coconut yogurt
- 1/2 cup granola
- 1/2 cup mixed berries (strawberries, blueberries, raspberries)
- 2 tablespoons shredded coconut
- 1 tablespoon honey or maple syrup (optional)
- Fresh mint leaves for garnish (optional)

Instructions:

1. In a serving glass or bowl, start by layering a portion of coconut yogurt at the bottom.
2. Add a layer of granola on top of the coconut yogurt.
3. Scatter a handful of mixed berries over the granola layer.
4. Repeat the layers until you reach the top of the glass or bowl.

5. Drizzle honey or maple syrup over the top layer for added sweetness, if desired.

6. Finish by sprinkling shredded coconut over the parfait.

7. Garnish with fresh mint leaves for a burst of freshness.

8. Serve immediately and enjoy your delicious and nutritious Coconut Yogurt Parfait!

Homemade Almond Butter Cups:

Ingredients:

- 1 cup dark chocolate chips or chopped dark chocolate
- 1/2 cup almond butter
- 2 tablespoons coconut oil
- 2 tablespoons maple syrup or honey
- 1/2 teaspoon vanilla extract
- A pinch of salt (optional)

Instructions:

1. Line a mini muffin tin with paper or silicone liners.

2. In a heatproof bowl, melt the dark chocolate and 1 tablespoon of coconut oil together using a microwave or a double boiler. Stir until smooth.

3. Spoon a small amount of melted chocolate into the bottom of each cup, spreading it to coat the bottom and slightly up the sides.

4. Place the muffin tin in the freezer for about 10-15 minutes to set the chocolate.

5. In a separate bowl, mix almond butter, remaining coconut oil, maple syrup or honey, vanilla extract, and a pinch of salt if desired.

6. Remove the muffin tin from the freezer and spoon a small amount of the almond butter mixture into each cup, spreading it to cover the chocolate layer.

7. Pour the remaining melted chocolate over the almond butter layer, covering it completely.

8. Place the muffin tin back in the freezer and let the almond butter cups set for at least 30 minutes.

9. Once set, remove the almond butter cups from the freezer. Peel off the liners.

10. Store the Homemade Almond Butter Cups in the refrigerator.

11. Enjoy these delicious and healthier treats.

Orange and Pistachio Quinoa Pudding:

Ingredients:

- 1 cup cooked quinoa
- 2 cups milk (dairy or plant-based)
- Zest of 1 orange
- 1/4 cup fresh orange juice
- 1/4 cup honey or maple syrup
- 1/2 teaspoon vanilla extract
- 1/4 teaspoon ground cinnamon
- 1/4 cup chopped pistachios
- Fresh orange segments for garnish

Instructions:

1. In a saucepan, combine cooked quinoa, milk, orange zest, fresh orange juice, honey or maple syrup, vanilla extract, and ground cinnamon.

2. Place the saucepan over medium heat and bring the mixture to a gentle simmer.

3. Reduce the heat to low and let the quinoa pudding simmer for about 15-20 minutes, stirring occasionally, until it thickens.

4. Stir in the chopped pistachios during the last few minutes of cooking.

5. Once the quinoa pudding has reached your desired consistency, remove it from the heat.

6. Let the pudding cool slightly before serving. It will continue to thicken as it cools.

7. Spoon the Orange and Pistachio Quinoa Pudding into serving bowls.

8. Garnish with fresh orange segments and additional chopped pistachios if desired.

9. Serve warm or chilled, and enjoy this unique and flavorful quinoa pudding!

CHAPTER 7: BEVERAGES ALIGNED WITH BLOOD TYPE O POSITIVE DIET

Green Tea:

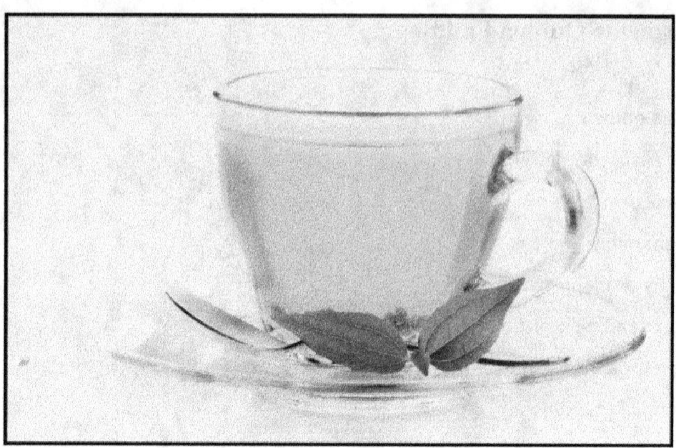

Ingredients:

- 1 teaspoon green tea leaves or 1 green tea bag
- 1 cup water (heated to about 175°F or 80°C)
- Optional: Honey or lemon for sweetening

Instructions:

1. Boil water and let it cool for a minute to reach the optimal temperature for green tea (around 175°F or 80°C).
2. Place green tea leaves in a teapot or tea infuser if using loose leaves. If using a tea bag, simply place it in your cup.
3. Pour the hot water over the green tea leaves or tea bag.
4. Steep the green tea for 2-3 minutes. Steeping too long may result in a bitter taste, so adjust based on your preference.
5. Remove the tea leaves or bag from the water.
6. Optional: Add honey or a slice of lemon to enhance the flavor.

7. Stir gently and enjoy your freshly brewed Green Tea!

Water with Lemon:

Ingredients:

- 1 glass of water (8-12 ounces)
- 1/2 lemon, sliced

Instructions:

1. Fill a glass with water.
2. Slice half a lemon into thin rounds or wedges.
3. Squeeze the juice from a few lemon slices into the water if you prefer a stronger lemon flavor.
4. Drop the lemon slices into the water.
5. Allow the water to sit for a few minutes to infuse with the lemon flavor.
6. Optionally, add ice cubes if you prefer a chilled beverage.
7. Stir gently and enjoy your refreshing and hydrating Water with Lemon!

Ginger Tea:

Ingredients:

- 1-inch piece of fresh ginger, peeled and sliced
- 1 cup water
- Honey or lemon (optional, for flavor)
- Fresh mint leaves (optional, for garnish)

Instructions:

1. Peel and thinly slice the fresh ginger, ensuring it's about a 1-inch piece.
2. Bring 1 cup of water to a boil in a small saucepan.
3. Add the sliced ginger to the boiling water.
4. Reduce the heat to low, cover the saucepan, and let it simmer for about 5-10 minutes, depending on how strong you prefer the ginger flavor.
5. If desired, add honey or a squeeze of lemon for extra flavor. Stir to combine.

6. Strain the ginger tea into a cup, removing the ginger slices.

7. Optional: Garnish with fresh mint leaves for a refreshing touch.

8. Allow the tea to cool for a few minutes before sipping.

9. Enjoy your soothing and invigorating Ginger Tea!

Berry Smoothie with Almond Milk:

Ingredients:
- 1 cup mixed berries (strawberries, blueberries, raspberries)
- 1 banana, peeled and sliced
- 1 cup almond milk (unsweetened)
- 1/2 cup Greek yogurt (optional for added creaminess)
- 1 tablespoon honey or maple syrup (optional for sweetness)
- Ice cubes (optional)
- Chia seeds or flax seeds for garnish (optional)

Instructions:
1. In a blender, combine the mixed berries, sliced banana, almond milk, and Greek yogurt if using.
2. Optional: Add honey or maple syrup for sweetness.
3. If you prefer a colder smoothie, add a handful of ice cubes to the blender.
4. Blend the ingredients on high speed until the mixture is smooth and creamy.
5. Taste the smoothie and adjust sweetness or thickness by adding more honey, maple syrup, or almond milk as needed.
6. Pour the Berry Smoothie into glasses.
7. Optional: Garnish with a sprinkle of chia seeds or flaxseeds for added texture and nutrition.
8. Serve immediately and enjoy your delicious and nutritious Berry Smoothie with Almond Milk!

Herbal Mint Tea:

Ingredients:
- 1 cup fresh mint leaves (or 1-2 tablespoons dried mint leaves)
- 1 teaspoon dried chamomile flowers (optional)
- 1 teaspoon dried lavender flowers (optional)
- 1 cup water

- Honey or lemon for flavor (optional)

Instructions:

1. Rinse the fresh mint leaves under cold water.
2. If using dried herbs, measure out the dried mint leaves, chamomile flowers, and lavender flowers.
3. In a teapot or heat proof container, place the fresh mint leaves or dried herbs.
4. Boil 1 cup of water.
5. Pour the boiling water over the mint leaves or dried herbs in the teapot.
6. Let the herbal mixture steep for 5-7 minutes, or longer for a stronger flavor.
7. Optional: Add honey or a squeeze of lemon for extra flavor. Stir to combine.
8. Strain the Herbal Mint Tea into a cup to remove the leaves or herbs.
9. Allow the tea to cool slightly before sipping.
10. Enjoy the soothing and aromatic experience of Herbal Mint Tea!

Pineapple and Turmeric Smoothie:

Ingredients:
- 1 cup pineapple chunks (fresh or frozen)
- 1 banana, peeled
- 1/2 teaspoon ground turmeric
- 1/2 teaspoon fresh ginger, grated
- 1 cup coconut water or almond milk
- 1 tablespoon chia seeds (optional)
- Ice cubes (optional)
- Honey or maple syrup for sweetness (optional)

Instructions:

1. In a blender, combine pineapple chunks, banana, ground turmeric, grated ginger, and coconut water or almond milk.
2. If you prefer a colder smoothie, add ice cubes to the blender.
3. Optional: Add chia seeds for extra fiber and nutrition.
4. Blend the ingredients on high speed until the smoothie reaches a creamy consistency.
5. Taste the smoothie and add honey or maple syrup if you desire additional sweetness.

6. Pour the Pineapple and Turmeric Smoothie into glasses.

7. Optional: Garnish with a slice of pineapple or a sprinkle of chia seeds for visual appeal.

8. Serve immediately and enjoy your vibrant and nutritious Pineapple and Turmeric Smoothie!

Watermelon Juice:

Ingredients:

- 4 cups seedless watermelon, cubed
- 1 tablespoon fresh lime or lemon juice (optional)
- Ice cubes (optional)
- Mint leaves for garnish (optional)

Instructions:

1. Cut the seedless watermelon into small, manageable cubes.

2. Place the watermelon cubes in a blender.

3. Optionally, add fresh lime or lemon juice for a hint of citrus flavor.

4. Blend the watermelon until it reaches a smooth consistency.

5. If you prefer a colder drink, add ice cubes to the blender and blend until the ice is crushed and well incorporated.

6. Strain the watermelon juice through a fine-mesh sieve or cheesecloth if you want a smoother texture (optional).

7. Pour the watermelon juice into glasses.

8. Optional: Garnish with mint leaves for a refreshing touch.

9. Serve immediately and enjoy your cool and hydrating Watermelon Juice!

Matcha Latte with Coconut Milk:

Ingredients:

- 1 teaspoon matcha powder
- 1 tablespoon hot water
- 1 cup coconut milk (or any milk of your choice)

- 1-2 teaspoons honey or sweetener of choice (optional)
- Ice cubes (for iced matcha latte, optional)

Instructions:

1. In a bowl, sift the matcha powder to avoid lumps.
2. Add one tablespoon of hot water to the matcha powder in the bowl.
3. Whisk the matcha and hot water together until it forms a smooth, vibrant green paste.
4. In a separate saucepan, heat the coconut milk until it's warm but not boiling.
5. If desired, add honey or sweetener to the warmed coconut milk and stir until dissolved.
6. Pour the warm sweetened coconut milk over the matcha paste.
7. Whisk the matcha and coconut milk mixture until frothy. You can use a bamboo whisk or a regular whisk.
8. If making an iced matcha latte, pour the matcha mixture over ice cubes.
9. Optional: Dust the top of your matcha latte with a little extra matcha powder for presentation.
10. Enjoy your delicious and energizing Matcha Latte with Coconut Milk!

Cranberry Kombucha:

Ingredients:

- 1 gallon brewed and cooled black or green tea (about 4-6 tea bags)
- 1 cup sugar
- 1 cup cranberry juice (100% pure)
- 2 cups kombucha from a previous batch (starter tea)
- Kombucha SCOBY (Symbiotic Culture Of Bacteria and Yeast)

Instructions:

1. Brew a gallon of tea using black or green tea bags. Let it steep for 15 minutes and then remove the tea bags.
2. While the tea is still warm, dissolve the sugar in it. Stir until the sugar is completely dissolved.
3. Allow the sweetened tea to cool to room temperature.
4. Once the tea is cool, transfer it to a large, clean glass jar.

5. Add the cranberry juice to the jar.

6. Add the kombucha SCOBY and the 2 cups of kombucha from a previous batch (starter tea).

7. Cover the jar with a clean cloth or coffee filter and secure it with a rubber band. This allows airflow while preventing debris from entering.

8. Place the jar in a dark and warm location, away from direct sunlight.

9. Allow the kombucha to ferment for 7-14 days. Taste it periodically until it reaches your desired level of tanginess.

10. Once the fermentation is complete, remove the SCOBY and reserve it along with some liquid for your next batch.

11. Strain the cranberry kombucha to remove any remaining solids.

12. Bottle the kombucha in airtight bottles, leaving about an inch of headspace.

13. Optional: Allow the bottled kombucha to carbonate by leaving it at room temperature for an additional 2-5 days.

14. Refrigerate the cranberry kombucha to stop the fermentation process.

15. Serve chilled, and enjoy your homemade Cranberry Kombucha!

Dandelion Root Coffee:

Ingredients:

- 2 tablespoons roasted dandelion root (ground)
- 1 cup water
- Plant-based milk (optional)
- Sweetener of choice (optional)

Instructions:

1. Bring 1 cup of water to a boil.

2. Place 2 tablespoons of ground roasted dandelion root in a heatproof container or teapot.

3. Pour the boiling water over the dandelion root.

4. Let the dandelion root steep for 5-10 minutes, depending on how strong you want your "coffee."

5. Strain the liquid to remove the dandelion root particles.

6. Optionally, add plant-based milk for creaminess and a sweetener of your choice if desired.

7. Stir well and adjust the sweetness to your liking.

8. Serve your Dandelion Root Coffee hot and enjoy this caffeine-free alternative!

Golden Milk Latte:

Ingredients:

- 1 cup milk of your choice (dairy or plant-based)
- 1 teaspoon ground turmeric
- 1/2 teaspoon ground cinnamon
- 1/4 teaspoon ground ginger
- A pinch of black pepper
- 1 tablespoon honey or maple syrup (adjust to taste)
- 1 tablespoon coconut oil (optional)
- A dash of vanilla extract (optional)

Instructions:

1. In a small saucepan, heat the milk over medium heat until it's warm but not boiling.

2. Add ground turmeric, ground cinnamon, ground ginger, a pinch of black pepper, honey or maple syrup, and coconut oil (if using) to the warm milk.

3. Whisk the ingredients together thoroughly while heating. Adjust sweetness to taste.

4. Continue to heat and whisk the mixture until it's well-combined and warmed through.

5. Optional: Add a dash of vanilla extract for additional flavor.

6. Once the Golden Milk Latte is well-blended and heated to your liking, remove it from the heat.

7. Pour the golden milk into a mug.

8. Stir once more before serving to ensure the spices are evenly distributed.

CHAPTER 8: SPECIAL OCCASION AND CELEBRATION RECIPES

Grilled Lemon Herb Chicken:

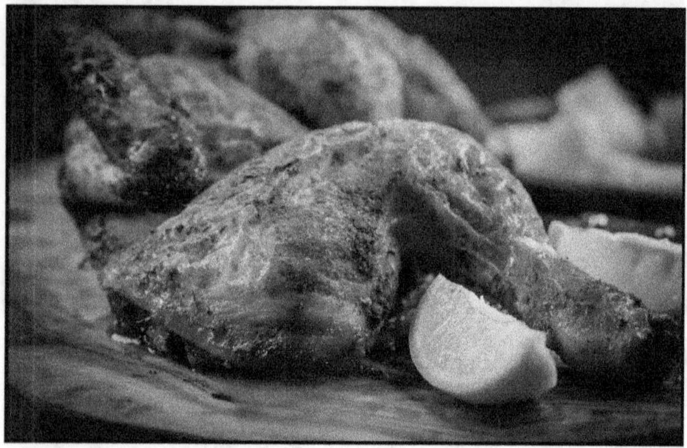

Ingredients:

- 4 boneless, skinless chicken breasts
- 2 lemons, juiced
- 3 tablespoons olive oil
- 2 cloves garlic, minced
- 1 teaspoon dried oregano
- 1 teaspoon dried thyme
- 1 teaspoon dried rosemary
- Salt and pepper to taste

Instructions:

1. In a bowl, combine lemon juice, olive oil, minced garlic, oregano, thyme, rosemary, salt, and pepper to create the marinade.

2. Place chicken breasts in a resealable plastic bag or shallow dish and pour the marinade over them. Ensure each piece is well-coated. Marinate in the refrigerator for at least 30 minutes, or ideally, overnight for more flavor.

3. Preheat the grill to medium-high heat.

4. Remove chicken from the marinade, letting excess drip off, and place on the preheated grill.

5. Grill the chicken for about 6-8 minutes per side or until the internal temperature reaches 165°F (74°C) and the chicken is no longer pink in the center.

6. While grilling, you can baste the chicken with any remaining marinade for added flavor.

7. Once cooked, remove the chicken from the grill and let it rest for a few minutes before serving.

8. Garnish with fresh herbs or lemon slices if desired. Enjoy your Grilled Lemon Herb Chicken!

Mango Avocado Salsa:

Ingredients:

- 1 ripe mango, peeled, pitted, and diced
- 1 ripe avocado, peeled, pitted, and diced
- 1/2 red onion, finely chopped
- 1 small jalapeño, seeds removed and finely chopped
- 1/4 cup fresh cilantro, chopped
- Juice of 1 lime
- Salt and pepper to taste

Instructions:

1. In a mixing bowl, combine diced mango, diced avocado, chopped red onion, jalapeño, and cilantro.

2. Squeeze fresh lime juice over the mixture to add a zesty flavor. Adjust the amount based on your taste preferences.

3. Gently toss the ingredients together until well combined.

4. Season the salsa with salt and pepper to taste. Mix again to ensure the flavors are evenly distributed.

5. Cover the bowl with plastic wrap and refrigerate for at least 30 minutes to allow the flavors to meld.

6. Before serving, give the salsa a final gentle stir. Adjust lime, salt, or pepper if needed.

7. Serve the Mango Avocado Salsa as a refreshing topping for grilled chicken, fish, tacos, or enjoy it with tortilla chips.

8. Garnish with additional cilantro if desired. Enjoy your vibrant and delicious Mango Avocado Salsa!

Stuffed Portobello Mushrooms:

Ingredients:

- 4 large portobello mushrooms, stems removed
- 1 cup breadcrumbs
- 1/2 cup grated Parmesan cheese
- 1/2 cup shredded mozzarella cheese
- 1/4 cup fresh parsley, chopped
- 2 cloves garlic, minced
- 2 tablespoons olive oil
- Salt and pepper to taste
- Optional: Cherry tomatoes for garnish

Instructions:

1. Preheat the oven to 375°F (190°C).

2. Clean the portobello mushrooms and remove the stems. Place the mushrooms on a baking sheet, gill side up.

3. In a bowl, combine breadcrumbs, Parmesan cheese, mozzarella cheese, chopped parsley, minced garlic, olive oil, salt, and pepper. Mix until well combined.

4. Stuff each portobello mushroom cap with the breadcrumb mixture, pressing it down gently.

5. Optional: Garnish the stuffed mushrooms with halved cherry tomatoes for extra flavor and color.

6. Bake in the preheated oven for 20-25 minutes or until the mushrooms are tender and the topping is golden brown.

7. Remove from the oven and let them cool for a few minutes before serving.

8. Serve the Stuffed Portobello Mushrooms as a delightful appetizer or a side dish. Enjoy the savory goodness!

Shrimp Scampi Pasta:

Ingredients:

- 8 oz (about 225g) linguine or your preferred pasta
- 1 lb (about 450g) large shrimp, peeled and deveined
- 4 tablespoons unsalted butter
- 4 tablespoons olive oil
- 4 cloves garlic, minced
- 1/2 teaspoon red pepper flakes (adjust to taste)
- 1/2 cup dry white wine
- Juice of 1 lemon
- Salt and black pepper to taste
- Fresh parsley, chopped, for garnish
- Grated Parmesan cheese for serving

Instructions:

1. Cook the pasta according to package instructions until al dente. Drain and set aside.

2. In a large skillet, heat 2 tablespoons of butter and 2 tablespoons of olive oil over medium heat.

3. Add minced garlic and red pepper flakes, sautéing for about 1 minute until the garlic is fragrant.

4. Add the shrimp to the skillet, cooking for 2-3 minutes on each side until they turn pink and opaque. Season with salt and black pepper.

5. Remove the shrimp from the skillet and set them aside.

6. In the same skillet, add the white wine and lemon juice, scraping any browned bits from the bottom of the pan. Simmer for 2-3 minutes to reduce the liquid slightly.

7. Stir in the remaining 2 tablespoons of butter and 2 tablespoons of olive oil until melted.

8. Add the cooked pasta and shrimp back to the skillet, tossing everything together to coat in the flavorful sauce.

9. Adjust salt and pepper to taste. If the sauce is too thick, you can add a splash of pasta cooking water to reach your desired consistency.

10. Garnish with chopped fresh parsley and serve the Shrimp Scampi Pasta hot, with grated Parmesan cheese on the side. Enjoy this delicious and classic dish!

Baked Salmon with Dill Sauce:

Ingredients:

- 4 salmon fillets (about 6 oz each)
- 2 tablespoons olive oil
- Salt and black pepper to taste
- 1 lemon, thinly sliced (for garnish)

For Dill Sauce:

- 1/2 cup plain Greek yogurt
- 2 tablespoons mayonnaise
- 1 tablespoon Dijon mustard
- 1 tablespoon fresh dill, chopped
- 1 clove garlic, minced
- 1 tablespoon lemon juice

- Salt and black pepper to taste

Instructions:

1. Preheat the oven to 375°F (190°C).
2. Place salmon fillets on a baking sheet lined with parchment paper. Drizzle olive oil over the fillets and season with salt and black pepper.
3. Arrange lemon slices on top of the salmon fillets for added flavor.
4. Bake in the preheated oven for 15-20 minutes or until the salmon is cooked through and easily flakes with a fork.
5. While the salmon is baking, prepare the dill sauce. In a bowl, combine Greek yogurt, mayonnaise, Dijon mustard, chopped dill, minced garlic, and lemon juice. Mix until well combined.
6. Season the dill sauce with salt and black pepper to taste. Adjust the ingredients as needed for your preferred flavor.
7. Once the salmon is done, remove it from the oven and transfer the filets to serving plates.
8. Drizzle the dill sauce over the baked salmon or serve it on the side.
9. Garnish with additional fresh dill and lemon slices if desired.
10. Serve the Baked Salmon with Dill Sauce alongside your favorite side dishes. Enjoy a flavorful and healthy meal!

Quinoa Salad with Pomegranate and Feta:

Ingredients:

- 1 cup quinoa, rinsed and cooked according to package instructions
- 1 cup pomegranate arils (seeds)
- 1/2 cup crumbled feta cheese
- 1/2 cup cucumber, diced
- 1/4 cup red onion, finely chopped
- 1/4 cup fresh parsley, chopped
- 2 tablespoons extra-virgin olive oil

- 1 tablespoon balsamic vinegar
- Salt and black pepper to taste

Instructions:

1. Cook the quinoa according to package instructions. Once cooked, allow it to cool to room temperature.
2. In a large bowl, combine the cooled quinoa, pomegranate arils, crumbled feta cheese, diced cucumber, chopped red onion, and fresh parsley.
3. In a small bowl, whisk together the extra-virgin olive oil and balsamic vinegar to create the dressing.
4. Drizzle the dressing over the quinoa mixture and toss gently until all ingredients are well coated.
5. Season the salad with salt and black pepper to taste. Adjust seasoning as needed.
6. Refrigerate the Quinoa Salad for at least 30 minutes before serving to allow the flavors to meld.
7. Before serving, give the salad a final toss and garnish with additional fresh parsley, if desired.
8. Serve the Quinoa Salad with Pomegranate and Feta as a refreshing and nutritious side dish or a light meal. Enjoy!

Lemon Rosemary Roasted Potatoes:

Ingredients:

- 1.5 lbs (about 700g) baby potatoes, halved or quartered
- 3 tablespoons olive oil
- Zest of 1 lemon
- Juice of 1 lemon
- 2 tablespoons fresh rosemary, chopped
- 3 cloves garlic, minced
- Salt and black pepper to taste

Instructions:

1. Preheat the oven to 425°F (220°C).

2. In a large bowl, combine halved or quartered baby potatoes, olive oil, lemon zest, lemon juice, chopped rosemary, and minced garlic.

3. Toss the potatoes in the mixture until they are evenly coated with the seasonings.

4. Season with salt and black pepper to taste, ensuring the potatoes are well-seasoned.

5. Spread the potatoes in a single layer on a baking sheet lined with parchment paper or a silicone baking mat.

6. Roast in the preheated oven for 25-30 minutes or until the potatoes are golden brown and crispy on the edges, flipping them halfway through for even cooking.

7. Once done, remove from the oven and transfer the Lemon Rosemary Roasted Potatoes to a serving dish.

8. Garnish with additional chopped rosemary and lemon zest if desired.

9. Serve as a delicious side dish alongside your favorite main course. Enjoy the zesty and aromatic flavors of these roasted potatoes!

Caprese Stuffed Chicken Breast:

Ingredients:

- 4 boneless, skinless chicken breasts
- 1 cup cherry tomatoes, halved
- 4 ounces fresh mozzarella cheese, sliced
- 1/4 cup fresh basil leaves, thinly sliced
- 2 tablespoons balsamic glaze
- Salt and black pepper to taste
- 2 tablespoons olive oil

Instructions:

1. Preheat the oven to 400°F (200°C).

2. Butterfly each chicken breast by cutting horizontally, but not all the way through, so you can open it like a book.

3. Season the inside of each chicken breast with salt and black pepper.

4. Place halved cherry tomatoes, sliced fresh mozzarella, and thinly sliced basil inside each butterflied chicken breast.

5. Close the chicken breasts and secure with toothpicks, if needed, to keep the stuffing in place.

6. Heat olive oil in an oven-safe skillet over medium-high heat.

7. Sear the stuffed chicken breasts for 2-3 minutes on each side until golden brown.

8. Transfer the skillet to the preheated oven and bake for 20-25 minutes or until the chicken reaches an internal temperature of 165°F (74°C).

9. During the last few minutes of baking, you can place additional slices of mozzarella on top of each chicken breast to melt.

10. Once cooked, drizzle balsamic glaze over the Caprese Stuffed Chicken Breasts before serving.

11. Remove toothpicks before serving and garnish with extra basil if desired.

12. Serve these flavorful and cheesy chicken breasts with your favorite side dishes. Enjoy your Caprese Stuffed Chicken!

Chocolate Avocado Mousse:

Ingredients:

- 2 ripe avocados, peeled and pitted
- 1/2 cup cocoa powder
- 1/2 cup maple syrup or agave nectar
- 1/4 cup almond milk or any preferred milk
- 1 teaspoon vanilla extract
- Pinch of salt
- Optional toppings: Fresh berries, chopped nuts, or whipped coconut cream

Instructions:

1. In a blender or food processor, combine ripe avocados, cocoa powder, maple syrup, almond milk, vanilla extract, and a pinch of salt.

2. Blend the ingredients until smooth and creamy, scraping down the sides as needed to ensure everything is well combined.

3. Taste the chocolate avocado mixture and adjust the sweetness if necessary by adding more maple syrup or agave nectar.

4. Once the mousse reaches a smooth consistency, spoon it into serving glasses or bowls.

5. Refrigerate the Chocolate Avocado Mousse for at least 2 hours to allow it to set and chill.

6. Before serving, garnish with fresh berries, chopped nuts, or a dollop of whipped coconut cream if desired.

7. Serve chilled and enjoy this rich and indulgent chocolate dessert that's secretly healthy with the goodness of avocados!

Raspberry Almond Tart:

Ingredients:

For the Crust:

- 1 1/2 cups all-purpose flour
- 1/2 cup almond flour
- 1/2 cup unsalted butter, cold and cubed
- 1/4 cup granulated sugar
- 1/4 teaspoon salt
- 1 large egg, beaten

For the Almond Cream Filling:

- 1/2 cup unsalted butter, softened
- 1/2 cup granulated sugar
- 1 cup almond flour
- 2 large eggs
- 1 teaspoon almond extract

For Topping:

- 2 cups fresh raspberries
- Powdered sugar for dusting

Instructions:

1. Preheat the oven to 375°F (190°C).
2. For the crust, in a food processor, combine all-purpose flour, almond flour, cold cubed butter, granulated sugar, and salt. Pulse until the mixture resembles coarse crumbs.
3. Add the beaten egg and pulse until the dough comes together. Form the dough into a ball, flatten it into a disk, wrap in plastic wrap, and refrigerate for at least 30 minutes.
4. Roll out the chilled dough on a floured surface and transfer it to a tart pan. Press the dough into the pan, ensuring an even layer on the bottom and up the sides. Trim any excess dough.
5. For the almond cream filling, beat together softened butter and granulated sugar until light and fluffy. Add almond flour, eggs, and almond extract. Mix until smooth.
6. Spread the almond cream filling evenly over the prepared tart crust.
7. Bake in the preheated oven for 20-25 minutes or until the crust is golden brown and the almond filling is set.
8. Allow the tart to cool completely before adding the raspberry topping.
9. Arrange fresh raspberries on top of the almond filling.
10. Dust the tart with powdered sugar just before serving.
11. Slice and enjoy your Raspberry Almond Tart with its delightful combination of almond cream, fresh raspberries, and buttery crust!

Caramelized Onion and Goat Cheese Crostini:

Ingredients:

- Baguette, thinly sliced
- 2 large onions, thinly sliced

- 2 tablespoons olive oil
- 1 tablespoon balsamic vinegar
- 1 teaspoon sugar
- Salt and black pepper to taste
- 4 ounces (about 113g) goat cheese
- Fresh thyme leaves for garnish (optional)

Instructions:

1. Preheat the oven to 375°F (190°C).
2. Place the baguette slices on a baking sheet and toast them in the preheated oven for 5-7 minutes or until golden and crisp.
3. In a skillet, heat olive oil over medium heat. Add thinly sliced onions and cook, stirring occasionally, until they start to soften.
4. Sprinkle sugar over the onions and continue cooking, stirring occasionally, until the onions caramelize and turn golden brown. This process may take about 15-20 minutes.
5. Deglaze the pan with balsamic vinegar, scraping up any browned bits. Cook for an additional 2-3 minutes until the vinegar has evaporated.
6. Season the caramelized onions with salt and black pepper to taste.
7. Spread a layer of goat cheese on each toasted baguette slice.
8. Top the goat cheese with a generous spoonful of the caramelized onions.
9. Optional: Garnish with fresh thyme leaves for added flavor and presentation.
10. Arrange the Caramelized Onion and Goat Cheese Crostini on a serving platter and serve immediately as a delicious appetizer or snack. Enjoy the sweet and savory combination!

CHAPTER 9: BLOOD TYPE O POSITIVE WEEKLY MEAL PLAN

Day 1:

Breakfast: Omelette with spinach and tomatoes

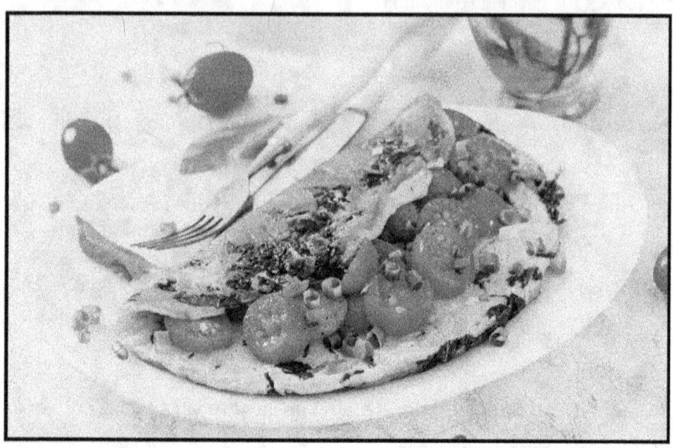

Ingredients:

- 3 large eggs
- 1/4 cup milk
- Salt and black pepper to taste
- 1 tablespoon butter or cooking oil
- 1 cup fresh spinach, chopped
- 1/2 cup cherry tomatoes, halved
- 1/4 cup shredded cheese (cheddar, feta, or your choice)

Instructions:

1. In a bowl, whisk together eggs, milk, salt, and black pepper until well combined.
2. Heat butter or cooking oil in a non-stick skillet over medium heat.
3. Add chopped spinach to the skillet and sauté until wilted.

4. Pour the whisked egg mixture over the spinach in the skillet.

5. Allow the eggs to set slightly at the edges, and then gently lift the edges with a spatula, tilting the skillet to let the uncooked eggs flow to the edges.

6. Once the omelette is mostly set but still slightly runny on top, add halved cherry tomatoes and sprinkle shredded cheese over one half of the omelette.

7. Carefully fold the other half of the omelette over the tomatoes and cheese, creating a half-moon shape.

8. Cook for an additional 1-2 minutes until the cheese melts and the omelette is cooked through.

9. Slide the omelet onto a plate and garnish with additional salt, pepper, or herbs if desired.

10. Serve your Spinach and Tomato Omelette hot, accompanied by toast or your favorite breakfast sides. Enjoy a nutritious and flavorful start to your day!

Snack: Apple slices with almond butter

Ingredients:

- 2 apples, cored and sliced
- 1/4 cup almond butter
- Optional toppings: Chia seeds, honey, or cinnamon

Instructions:

1. Core and slice the apples into thin wedges.

2. Spread a layer of almond butter on each apple slice.

3. Optional: Drizzle honey over the almond butter or sprinkle chia seeds or cinnamon for added flavor and texture.

4. Arrange the apple slices on a serving plate.

5. Serve the Apple Slices with Almond Butter as a quick and healthy snack. Enjoy the delightful combination of sweet, crunchy apples, and creamy almond butter!

Lunch: Grilled chicken salad with mixed greens

Ingredients:

For the Grilled Chicken:

- 2 boneless, skinless chicken breasts
- 2 tablespoons olive oil
- 1 teaspoon dried oregano
- 1 teaspoon garlic powder
- Salt and black pepper to taste

For the Salad:

- Mixed salad greens (e.g., spinach, arugula, lettuce)
- Cherry tomatoes, halved
- Cucumber, sliced
- Red bell pepper, sliced
- Red onion, thinly sliced
- Feta cheese, crumbled
- Kalamata olives (optional)

For the Dressing:

- 3 tablespoons extra-virgin olive oil
- 2 tablespoons balsamic vinegar
- 1 teaspoon Dijon mustard
- 1 teaspoon honey
- Salt and black pepper to taste

Instructions:

1. Preheat the grill or grill pan over medium-high heat.
2. In a bowl, combine olive oil, dried oregano, garlic powder, salt, and black pepper. Brush the mixture over the chicken breasts.
3. Grill the chicken breasts for 6-8 minutes per side or until fully cooked and juices run clear. Allow the chicken to rest for a few minutes before slicing.

4. In a large salad bowl, combine mixed salad greens, cherry tomatoes, cucumber, red bell pepper, red onion, feta cheese, and Kalamata olives if using.

5. Slice the grilled chicken into strips and place them on top of the salad.

6. In a small bowl, whisk together extra-virgin olive oil, balsamic vinegar, Dijon mustard, honey, salt, and black pepper to make the dressing.

7. Drizzle the dressing over the grilled chicken and salad.

8. Toss the salad gently to combine all the ingredients and coat them in the dressing.

9. Serve the Grilled Chicken Salad with Mixed Greens immediately. Enjoy a satisfying and flavorful lunch!

Snack: Greek yogurt with berries

Ingredients:

- 1 cup Greek yogurt
- 1/2 cup mixed berries (strawberries, blueberries, raspberries)
- 1 tablespoon honey
- Optional toppings: Granola, chia seeds, or mint leaves

Instructions:

1. Spoon Greek yogurt into a serving bowl.

2. Wash and prepare the mixed berries, then scatter them over the Greek yogurt.

3. Drizzle honey over the yogurt and berries for sweetness.

4. Optional: Sprinkle granola or chia seeds for added texture and nutritional benefits.

5. Garnish with fresh mint leaves if desired.

6. Serve the Greek Yogurt with Berries as a refreshing and nutritious snack. Enjoy the creamy yogurt paired with the natural sweetness of fresh berries!

Dinner: Salmon with sweet potato and steamed broccoli

Ingredients:

For the Salmon:

- 4 salmon fillets

- 2 tablespoons olive oil
- 1 tablespoon lemon juice
- 2 cloves garlic, minced
- 1 teaspoon dried dill
- Salt and black pepper to taste

For the Sweet Potatoes:

- 2 large sweet potatoes, peeled and diced
- 2 tablespoons olive oil
- 1 teaspoon smoked paprika
- Salt and black pepper to taste

For the Steamed Broccoli:

- 1 bunch broccoli, cut into florets
- Lemon wedges for serving

Instructions:

1. Preheat the oven to 400°F (200°C).
2. In a bowl, mix together olive oil, lemon juice, minced garlic, dried dill, salt, and black pepper for the salmon.
3. Place the salmon fillets on a baking sheet lined with parchment paper. Brush the salmon with the prepared mixture.
4. In a separate bowl, toss diced sweet potatoes with olive oil, smoked paprika, salt, and black pepper. Spread them on another baking sheet.
5. Roast both the salmon and sweet potatoes in the preheated oven for about 15-20 minutes or until the salmon is cooked through, and the sweet potatoes are tender.
6. While the salmon and sweet potatoes are roasting, steam the broccoli until it's vibrant and tender, about 5-7 minutes.
7. Once everything is cooked, plate the salmon fillets, sweet potatoes, and steamed broccoli.
8. Serve with a wedge of lemon for squeezing over the salmon.

9. Enjoy your wholesome and balanced dinner of Salmon with Sweet Potato and Steamed Broccoli!

Day 2:

Breakfast: Quinoa porridge with sliced banana

Ingredients:

- 1/2 cup quinoa, rinsed
- 1 cup milk (dairy or plant-based)
- 1/2 cup water
- 1 tablespoon maple syrup or honey
- 1/2 teaspoon vanilla extract
- Pinch of salt
- 1 ripe banana, sliced
- Optional toppings: Nuts, seeds, or a sprinkle of cinnamon

Instructions:

1. Rinse the quinoa under cold water.
2. In a saucepan, combine quinoa, milk, water, maple syrup or honey, vanilla extract, and a pinch of salt.
3. Bring the mixture to a boil, then reduce the heat to low, cover, and simmer for about 15-20 minutes or until the quinoa is cooked and the porridge has thickened.
4. Stir occasionally to prevent sticking and ensure even cooking.
5. Once the quinoa is cooked, remove the saucepan from heat.
6. Serve the quinoa porridge in bowls and top with sliced bananas.
7. Optional: Sprinkle nuts, seeds, or a bit of cinnamon over the porridge for added flavor and texture.
8. Enjoy your nutritious and filling Quinoa Porridge with Sliced Banana as a wholesome breakfast to start your day!

Snack: Carrot sticks with hummus

Ingredients:

- Fresh carrots, peeled and cut into sticks
- Hummus for dipping

Instructions:

1. Wash, peel, and cut fresh carrots into sticks.
2. Arrange the carrot sticks on a plate or in a portable container.
3. Serve with a side of hummus for dipping.
4. Dip the carrot sticks into the hummus and enjoy this healthy and satisfying snack.
5. Optionally, you can sprinkle a pinch of salt, black pepper, or paprika on the hummus for extra flavor.
6. Carrot sticks with hummus make a crunchy, nutritious snack that's perfect for any time of the day. Enjoy!

Lunch: Turkey and avocado wrap with lettuce

Ingredients:

- 4 whole-grain or spinach tortillas
- 1 pound (about 450g) cooked turkey breast, sliced
- 2 ripe avocados, sliced
- 1 cup cherry tomatoes, halved
- 1 cup lettuce leaves, shredded
- 1/2 cup Greek yogurt or mayonnaise
- 1 tablespoon Dijon mustard
- Salt and black pepper to taste

Instructions:

1. In a small bowl, mix Greek yogurt or mayonnaise with Dijon mustard. Season with salt and black pepper to taste. This will be the sauce for your wrap.
2. Lay out the tortillas on a flat surface.
3. Spread the sauce evenly over each tortilla.

4. Arrange slices of cooked turkey on the tortillas, leaving space at one end to fold.

5. Place avocado slices, cherry tomatoes, and shredded lettuce on top of the turkey.

6. Fold the sides of the tortillas and roll them tightly to form wraps.

7. If desired, secure the wraps with toothpicks or parchment paper for easier handling.

8. Slice each wrap in half diagonally for serving.

9. Serve your Turkey and Avocado Wraps with Lettuce as a delicious and balanced lunch option.

10. Enjoy the combination of lean turkey, creamy avocado, and crisp lettuce in this satisfying wrap!

Snack: Mixed nuts

Ingredients:

- 1 cup mixed nuts (almonds, walnuts, cashews, pecans, etc.)
- 1 tablespoon olive oil
- 1 teaspoon honey (optional)
- 1/2 teaspoon salt (adjust to taste)
- Optional: Sprinkle of cinnamon, paprika, or your preferred seasoning

Instructions:

1. Preheat the oven to 350°F (175°C).

2. In a bowl, toss the mixed nuts with olive oil until they are evenly coated.

3. If desired, drizzle honey over the nuts and toss again for a touch of sweetness.

4. Sprinkle salt over the nuts, adjusting to your taste preference.

5. Optional: Add a sprinkle of cinnamon, paprika, or your preferred seasoning for extra flavor.

6. Spread the seasoned nuts in a single layer on a baking sheet lined with parchment paper.

7. Bake in the preheated oven for 10-15 minutes, stirring halfway through, or until the nuts are golden and fragrant.

8. Remove from the oven and let the mixed nuts cool completely before serving.

9. Once cooled, transfer the mixed nuts to a bowl or store them in an airtight container for later.

10. Enjoy your flavorful and crunchy Mixed Nuts as a healthy and satisfying snack!

Dinner: Beef stir-fry with bell peppers and brown rice

Ingredients:

For the Beef Stir-Fry:

- 1 pound (about 450g) beef sirloin or flank steak, thinly sliced
- 2 tablespoons soy sauce
- 1 tablespoon oyster sauce
- 1 tablespoon hoisin sauce
- 1 tablespoon cornstarch
- 2 tablespoons vegetable oil, divided
- 3 cloves garlic, minced
- 1 tablespoon ginger, grated
- 2 bell peppers (assorted colors), thinly sliced
- 1 cup broccoli florets

For the Brown Rice:

- 1 cup brown rice
- 2 cups water
- Salt to taste

Instructions:

1. In a bowl, mix soy sauce, oyster sauce, hoisin sauce, and cornstarch. Add sliced beef and marinate for at least 15 minutes.

2. In a wok or large skillet, heat 1 tablespoon of vegetable oil over high heat.

3. Add marinated beef to the wok and stir-fry for 2-3 minutes or until browned. Remove the beef from the wok and set aside.

4. In the same wok, add another tablespoon of vegetable oil.

5. Add minced garlic and grated ginger to the wok, stir-frying for about 30 seconds until fragrant.

6. Add sliced bell peppers and broccoli to the wok. Stir-fry for 3-4 minutes or until vegetables are tender-crisp.

7. Return the cooked beef to the wok and toss everything together until well combined and heated through.

8. While preparing the stir-fry, cook brown rice according to package instructions. Add salt to taste.

9. Serve the Beef Stir-Fry with Bell Peppers over a bed of brown rice.

10. Enjoy your flavorful and nutritious Beef Stir-Fry with the perfect balance of protein, veggies, and whole grains for dinner!

Day 3:

Breakfast: Smoothie with kale, banana, and pineapple

Ingredients:

- 1 cup kale leaves, stems removed
- 1 ripe banana
- 1 cup fresh pineapple chunks
- 1/2 cup Greek yogurt
- 1/2 cup coconut water or water
- 1 tablespoon chia seeds (optional)
- Ice cubes (optional)

Instructions:

1. Wash and prepare the kale leaves by removing the stems.

2. In a blender, combine kale leaves, ripe banana, fresh pineapple chunks, Greek yogurt, and coconut water (or water).

3. Optional: Add chia seeds for extra nutrition and thickness.

4. If you prefer a colder smoothie, you can add a handful of ice cubes.

5. Blend all the ingredients until smooth and creamy.

6. Taste the smoothie and adjust the sweetness by adding more bananas if needed.

7. Pour the kale, banana, and pineapple smoothie into a glass.

8. Optionally, garnish with additional pineapple chunks or a slice of banana.

9. Enjoy your refreshing and nutrient-packed smoothie as a healthy breakfast option!

Snack: Cottage cheese with pineapple chunks

Ingredients:

- 1 cup cottage cheese
- 1/2 cup pineapple chunks (fresh or canned, drained)
- Honey or maple syrup for drizzling (optional)

Instructions:

1. In a bowl, scoop 1 cup of cottage cheese.

2. Add pineapple chunks to the cottage cheese.

3. Gently mix the cottage cheese and pineapple together.

4. Optional: Drizzle honey or maple syrup over the cottage cheese and pineapple for added sweetness.

5. Serve the Cottage Cheese with Pineapple Chunks as a quick and satisfying snack.

6. Enjoy the combination of creamy cottage cheese and the natural sweetness of pineapple!

Lunch: Lentil soup with a side of mixed vegetables

Ingredients:

For Lentil Soup:

- 1 cup dried lentils, rinsed and drained
- 1 onion, finely chopped
- 2 carrots, diced
- 2 celery stalks, diced
- 3 cloves garlic, minced

- 1 can (14 oz) diced tomatoes
- 6 cups vegetable or chicken broth
- 1 teaspoon ground cumin
- 1 teaspoon ground coriander
- 1 teaspoon smoked paprika
- Salt and black pepper to taste
- 2 tablespoons olive oil
- Fresh parsley for garnish (optional)
- Lemon wedges for serving

For Mixed Vegetables:

- Assorted vegetables (e.g., broccoli, bell peppers, zucchini), chopped
- Olive oil
- Salt and black pepper to taste

Instructions:

For Lentil Soup:

1. In a large pot, heat olive oil over medium heat. Add chopped onions, carrots, celery, and garlic. Sauté until vegetables are softened.
2. Add rinsed lentils, diced tomatoes, ground cumin, ground coriander, smoked paprika, salt, and black pepper. Stir to combine.
3. Pour in vegetable or chicken broth. Bring the soup to a boil, then reduce heat to low, cover, and simmer for about 25-30 minutes or until lentils are tender.
4. Adjust seasoning if needed. Garnish with fresh parsley if desired.
5. Serve the lentil soup hot with lemon wedges on the side.

For Mixed Vegetables:

1. Preheat the oven to 400°F (200°C).
2. Toss chopped vegetables with olive oil, salt, and black pepper.
3. Spread the vegetables on a baking sheet in a single layer.
4. Roast in the preheated oven for about 20-25 minutes or until the vegetables are tender and slightly browned, stirring halfway through.

5. Serve the lentil soup with a side of roasted mixed vegetables for a nutritious and satisfying lunch. Enjoy!

Snack: Hard-boiled eggs

Ingredients:

- Eggs (as many as desired)

Instructions:

1. Place the eggs in a single layer in a saucepan or pot.
2. Add enough water to the pot to cover the eggs by about an inch.
3. Place the pot on the stove over medium-high heat.
4. Once the water reaches a rolling boil, reduce the heat to low, cover the pot, and let the eggs simmer for about 9-12 minutes.
5. Remove the pot from the heat and immediately transfer the eggs to a bowl of ice water.
6. Allow the eggs to cool for at least 5 minutes in the ice water to make peeling easier.
7. Gently tap each egg on a hard surface to crack the shell, then peel off the shell.
8. Slice the hard-boiled eggs or enjoy them whole as a quick and protein-packed snack.
9. Sprinkle with a pinch of salt and black pepper if desired.
10. Hard-boiled eggs can be refrigerated for later or enjoyed immediately. They make a convenient and nutritious snack!

Dinner: Grilled shrimp with quinoa and asparagus

Ingredients:

For Grilled Shrimp:

- 1 pound (about 450g) large shrimp, peeled and deveined
- 2 tablespoons olive oil
- 2 cloves garlic, minced

- 1 teaspoon paprika

- 1 teaspoon cumin

- Salt and black pepper to taste

- Lemon wedges for serving

For Quinoa:

- 1 cup quinoa, rinsed

- 2 cups water or vegetable broth

- Salt to taste

For Asparagus:

- 1 bunch asparagus, ends trimmed

- 1 tablespoon olive oil

- Salt and black pepper to taste

Instructions:

For Grilled Shrimp:

1. In a bowl, mix together olive oil, minced garlic, paprika, cumin, salt, and black pepper.

2. Add peeled and deveined shrimp to the marinade, ensuring they are well coated. Let them marinate for at least 15 minutes.

3. Preheat the grill or grill pan over medium-high heat.

4. Thread the marinated shrimp onto skewers.

5. Grill the shrimp for 2-3 minutes per side or until they are opaque and cooked through.

6. Remove the shrimp skewers from the grill and squeeze fresh lemon juice over them before serving.

For Quinoa:

1. In a saucepan, combine rinsed quinoa and water or vegetable broth. Add salt to taste.

2. Bring to a boil, then reduce heat to low, cover, and simmer for 15-20 minutes or until quinoa is cooked and liquid is absorbed.

3. Fluff the quinoa with a fork.

For Asparagus:

1. Preheat the oven to 400°F (200°C).

2. Toss trimmed asparagus with olive oil, salt, and black pepper.

3. Roast in the preheated oven for about 10-12 minutes or until the asparagus is tender but still crisp.

To Serve:

1. Arrange a portion of cooked quinoa on each plate.

2. Top with grilled shrimp skewers.

3. Place roasted asparagus on the side.

4. Serve this Grilled Shrimp with Quinoa and Asparagus for a flavorful and well-balanced dinner. Enjoy!

Day 4:

Breakfast: Whole grain toast with avocado

Ingredients:

- Whole grain bread slices
- Ripe avocados
- Salt and black pepper to taste
- Optional toppings: Red pepper flakes, crushed garlic, poached or fried eggs, sliced tomatoes, or a squeeze of lemon juice

Instructions:

1. Toast whole grain bread slices to your desired level of crispiness.

2. While the bread is toasting, halve ripe avocados and remove the pits.

3. Scoop the avocado flesh into a bowl.

4. Mash the avocado with a fork until it reaches your preferred level of creaminess.

5. Season the mashed avocado with salt and black pepper to taste. Mix well.

6. Once the toast is ready, spread the mashed avocado evenly over the toasted bread slices.

7. Optional: Customize your avocado toast with additional toppings like red pepper flakes, crushed garlic, poached or fried eggs, sliced tomatoes, or a squeeze of lemon juice.

8. Serve the Whole Grain Toast with Avocado as a nutritious and delicious breakfast. Enjoy the creamy avocado on crunchy whole grain toast!

Snack: Orange slices

Ingredients:

- Fresh oranges

Instructions:

1. Wash the oranges thoroughly.

2. Slice off the top and bottom of each orange.

3. Stand the orange on one of the flat ends and carefully slice away the peel, following the curve of the fruit.

4. Once the orange is peeled, lay it on its side and slice into rounds or wedges.

5. Arrange the orange slices on a plate or in a bowl.

6. Serve the fresh Orange Slices as a refreshing and healthy snack.

7. Enjoy the natural sweetness and citrus burst of flavor!

Lunch: Tuna salad with mixed greens

Ingredients:

For the Tuna Salad:

- 2 cans (about 5 ounces each) tuna, drained
- 1/4 cup mayonnaise
- 1 tablespoon Dijon mustard
- 1 celery stalk, finely chopped
- 1/4 red onion, finely chopped

- Salt and black pepper to taste
- Optional: Lemon juice, chopped fresh parsley

For the Mixed Greens:

- Mixed salad greens (e.g., spinach, arugula, lettuce)
- Cherry tomatoes, halved
- Cucumber, sliced
- Avocado, sliced

Instructions:

For the Tuna Salad:

1. In a bowl, combine drained tuna, mayonnaise, Dijon mustard, chopped celery, and chopped red onion.
2. Mix the ingredients until well combined.
3. Season the tuna salad with salt and black pepper to taste.
4. Optional: Add a squeeze of fresh lemon juice and chopped fresh parsley for extra flavor.

For the Mixed Greens:

1. In a separate bowl, toss mixed salad greens, halved cherry tomatoes, sliced cucumber, and sliced avocado.
2. Optional: Drizzle with your favorite salad dressing.

To Serve:

1. Plate a generous portion of the mixed greens.
2. Spoon the tuna salad on top of the mixed greens.
3. Garnish with additional parsley or lemon slices if desired.
4. Serve your Tuna Salad with Mixed Greens as a wholesome and satisfying lunch. Enjoy the combination of protein-rich tuna and crisp, fresh greens!

Snack: Rice cakes with almond butter

Ingredients:

- Rice cakes

- Almond butter

Instructions:

1. Take rice cakes and place them on a clean surface or a plate.
2. Using a knife or a spoon, spread a generous layer of almond butter onto each rice cake.
3. Optionally, you can drizzle honey or sprinkle a pinch of cinnamon on top for added flavor.
4. Arrange the rice cakes with almond butter on a serving plate.
5. Enjoy your Rice Cakes with Almond Butter as a quick and satisfying snack. The combination of the crispy rice cake and creamy almond butter is delightful!

Dinner: Chicken and vegetable skewers with sweet potato wedges

Ingredients:

For Chicken and Vegetable Skewers:

- 1 pound (about 450g) boneless, skinless chicken breasts, cut into cubes
- 1 zucchini, sliced
- 1 bell pepper (any color), cut into chunks
- 1 red onion, cut into chunks
- Cherry tomatoes
- 2 tablespoons olive oil
- 2 cloves garlic, minced
- 1 teaspoon dried oregano
- 1 teaspoon smoked paprika
- Salt and black pepper to taste
- Wooden skewers, soaked in water for 30 minutes

For Sweet Potato Wedges:

- 2 large sweet potatoes, washed and cut into wedges
- 2 tablespoons olive oil
- 1 teaspoon paprika

- 1 teaspoon garlic powder
- Salt and black pepper to taste

Instructions:

For Chicken and Vegetable Skewers:

1. In a bowl, mix olive oil, minced garlic, dried oregano, smoked paprika, salt, and black pepper.
2. Add chicken cubes to the marinade and let them marinate for at least 15 minutes.
3. Thread marinated chicken, zucchini slices, bell pepper chunks, red onion chunks, and cherry tomatoes onto the soaked wooden skewers.
4. Preheat the grill or grill pan over medium-high heat.
5. Grill the skewers for about 10-15 minutes, turning occasionally, or until the chicken is fully cooked and vegetables are tender.

For Sweet Potato Wedges:

1. Preheat the oven to 425°F (220°C).
2. In a bowl, toss sweet potato wedges with olive oil, paprika, garlic powder, salt, and black pepper until evenly coated.
3. Spread the sweet potato wedges on a baking sheet in a single layer.
4. Roast in the preheated oven for about 25-30 minutes or until the sweet potatoes are golden and crispy, turning them halfway through.

To Serve:

1. Arrange the grilled Chicken and Vegetable Skewers on a plate.
2. Serve alongside the crispy Sweet Potato Wedges.
3. Enjoy this delicious and balanced dinner with a mix of protein, vegetables, and sweet potatoes!

Day 5:

Breakfast: Greek yogurt parfait with granola and berries

Ingredients:

- 1 cup Greek yogurt
- 1/2 cup granola
- 1/2 cup mixed berries (strawberries, blueberries, raspberries)
- Honey for drizzling (optional)

Instructions:

1. In a glass or bowl, start with a layer of Greek yogurt.
2. Add a layer of granola on top of the yogurt.
3. Scatter a portion of mixed berries over the granola.
4. Repeat the layers until you fill the glass or bowl, finishing with a final layer of berries on top.
5. Optional: Drizzle honey over the parfait for added sweetness.
6. Serve the Greek Yogurt Parfait with Granola and Berries immediately as a delicious and nutritious breakfast.
7. Enjoy the combination of creamy yogurt, crunchy granola, and the natural sweetness of fresh berries!

Snack: Celery sticks with peanut butter

Ingredients:

- Fresh celery stalks, washed and cut into sticks
- Peanut butter

Instructions:

1. Wash and cut fresh celery stalks into sticks.
2. Spread a layer of peanut butter on one side of each celery stick.
3. Arrange the Peanut Butter-filled Celery Sticks on a plate.
4. Optionally, you can sprinkle a pinch of salt or add raisins on top of the peanut butter for added flavor.
5. Enjoy this quick and nutritious Celery Sticks with Peanut Butter as a satisfying snack!

Lunch: Spinach and feta stuffed chicken breast with roasted Brussels sprouts

Ingredients:

For Spinach and Feta Stuffed Chicken Breast:

- 4 boneless, skinless chicken breasts
- 2 cups fresh spinach, chopped
- 1/2 cup feta cheese, crumbled
- 2 cloves garlic, minced
- 1 tablespoon olive oil
- Salt and black pepper to taste
- Toothpicks for securing

For Roasted Brussels Sprouts:

- 1 pound (about 450g) Brussels sprouts, trimmed and halved
- 2 tablespoons olive oil
- Salt and black pepper to taste
- Optional: Balsamic glaze for drizzling

Instructions:

For Spinach and Feta Stuffed Chicken Breast:

1. Preheat the oven to 375°F (190°C).
2. In a skillet, heat olive oil over medium heat. Add minced garlic and chopped spinach. Sauté until the spinach wilts.
3. Remove the skillet from heat and stir in crumbled feta cheese.
4. Butterfly each chicken breast by cutting horizontally through the thickest part, leaving one edge intact.
5. Open each chicken breast and season the inside with salt and black pepper.
6. Spoon the spinach and feta mixture onto one side of each butterflied chicken breast.
7. Fold the other half of the chicken breast over the stuffing and secure with toothpicks.

8. Place the stuffed chicken breasts in a baking dish.

9. Bake in the preheated oven for about 25-30 minutes or until the chicken is cooked through.

For Roasted Brussels Sprouts:

1. Preheat the oven to 400°F (200°C).

2. Toss halved Brussels sprouts with olive oil, salt, and black pepper.

3. Spread the Brussels sprouts on a baking sheet in a single layer.

4. Roast in the preheated oven for about 20-25 minutes or until the Brussels sprouts are golden and crispy, stirring halfway through.

To Serve:

1. Plate the Spinach and Feta Stuffed Chicken Breast.

2. Serve alongside the Roasted Brussels Sprouts.

3. Optional: Drizzle balsamic glaze over the Brussels sprouts for added flavor.

4. Enjoy this flavorful and balanced lunch with a combination of stuffed chicken and roasted vegetables!

Snack: Cherry tomatoes with mozzarella

Ingredients:

- Cherry tomatoes
- Fresh mozzarella balls (bocconcini or ciliegine)
- Fresh basil leaves
- Extra-virgin olive oil
- Balsamic glaze (optional)
- Salt and black pepper to taste

Instructions:

1. Wash cherry tomatoes and slice them in half.

2. Drain the fresh mozzarella balls if needed.

3. On toothpicks or small skewers, alternate threading cherry tomato halves, mozzarella balls, and fresh basil leaves.

4. Arrange the Tomato and Mozzarella Skewers on a serving plate.

5. Drizzle extra-virgin olive oil over the skewers.

6. Optionally, you can add a touch of balsamic glaze for extra flavor.

7. Sprinkle salt and black pepper to taste.

8. Serve the Cherry Tomatoes with Mozzarella Skewers as a delightful and refreshing snack.

9. Enjoy the combination of juicy tomatoes, creamy mozzarella, and aromatic basil!

Dinner: Quinoa bowl with black beans, corn, and salsa

Ingredients:

- 1 cup quinoa, rinsed
- 2 cups water or vegetable broth
- 1 can (15 oz) black beans, drained and rinsed
- 1 cup corn kernels (fresh, frozen, or canned)
- 1 cup salsa (store-bought or homemade)
- 1 avocado, sliced
- Fresh cilantro, chopped (for garnish)
- Lime wedges (for serving)
- Salt and black pepper to taste

Instructions:

1. In a saucepan, combine quinoa and water or vegetable broth. Bring to a boil, then reduce heat to low, cover, and simmer for 15-20 minutes or until quinoa is cooked and liquid is absorbed. Fluff with a fork.

2. While the quinoa is cooking, heat black beans and corn in a separate pan over medium heat until warmed through.

3. Once quinoa is cooked, divide it among serving bowls.

4. Top the quinoa with warmed black beans and corn.

5. Spoon salsa over the quinoa, beans, and corn.

6. Arrange sliced avocado on top of each bowl.

7. Garnish with chopped fresh cilantro.

8. Season with salt and black pepper to taste.

9. Serve the Quinoa Bowl with Black Beans, Corn, and Salsa with lime wedges on the side.

10. Mix everything together before enjoying this flavorful and nutritious dinner bowl!

Day 6:

Breakfast: Scrambled eggs with spinach and feta cheese

Ingredients:

- 4 large eggs
- 1 cup fresh spinach, chopped
- 1/2 cup feta cheese, crumbled
- 2 tablespoons butter or olive oil
- Salt and black pepper to taste
- Optional: Fresh herbs (such as parsley or dill) for garnish

Instructions:

1. In a bowl, whisk the eggs until well beaten. Season with salt and black pepper.

2. Heat butter or olive oil in a skillet over medium heat.

3. Add chopped spinach to the skillet and sauté until wilted.

4. Pour the whisked eggs over the spinach in the skillet.

5. Allow the eggs to set for a moment, then gently stir with a spatula.

6. As the eggs start to set, crumble the feta cheese over them.

7. Continue stirring the eggs until they are fully cooked but still moist.

8. Optional: Garnish with fresh herbs for added flavor.

9. Serve the Scrambled Eggs with Spinach and Feta Cheese hot and enjoy this nutritious and delicious breakfast!

Snack: Sliced mango

Ingredients:

- Fresh ripe mango

Instructions:

1. Wash the mango thoroughly.
2. Slice off the sides of the mango, avoiding the large pit in the center.
3. Using a knife, make cross-hatch cuts in each mango half without cutting through the skin.
4. Invert the mango halves to expose the cubes, or use a spoon to scoop out the mango cubes.
5. Alternatively, you can peel the mango and slice it into thin wedges.
6. Arrange the Sliced Mango on a plate.
7. Enjoy the sweet and juicy mango slices as a refreshing and healthy snack!

Lunch: Turkey burger with lettuce wrap and sweet potato fries

Ingredients:

For Turkey Burgers:

- 1 pound ground turkey
- 1/4 cup breadcrumbs
- 1 egg
- 1/4 cup onion, finely chopped
- 1 clove garlic, minced
- 1 teaspoon dried oregano
- Salt and black pepper to taste
- Olive oil for cooking

For Lettuce Wraps:

- Large lettuce leaves (e.g., iceberg or butter lettuce)

For Sweet Potato Fries:

- 2 large sweet potatoes, cut into fries

- 2 tablespoons olive oil
- 1 teaspoon paprika
- 1 teaspoon garlic powder
- Salt and black pepper to taste

Instructions:

For Turkey Burgers:

1. In a bowl, combine ground turkey, breadcrumbs, egg, chopped onion, minced garlic, dried oregano, salt, and black pepper.
2. Mix the ingredients until well combined.
3. Divide the mixture into equal portions and shape them into burger patties.
4. Heat olive oil in a skillet over medium heat.
5. Cook the turkey burgers for about 5-6 minutes per side or until fully cooked.

For Lettuce Wraps:

1. Wash and pat dry large lettuce leaves to use as wraps.
2. Place a cooked turkey burger on a lettuce leaf.
3. Optional: Add your favorite burger toppings such as tomato slices, pickles, or avocado.

For Sweet Potato Fries:

1. Preheat the oven to 425°F (220°C).
2. In a bowl, toss sweet potato fries with olive oil, paprika, garlic powder, salt, and black pepper until evenly coated.
3. Spread the sweet potato fries on a baking sheet in a single layer.
4. Roast in the preheated oven for about 20-25 minutes or until the fries are golden and crispy, stirring them halfway through.

To Serve:

1. Serve the Turkey Burgers in Lettuce Wraps with a side of Sweet Potato Fries.
2. Enjoy this wholesome and low-carb lunch option!

Snack: Walnuts

Ingredients:

- Fresh walnuts

Instructions:

1. Purchase fresh walnuts or store them in a cool, dry place.
2. If the walnuts are in the shell, crack and remove the shells.
3. Enjoy the walnuts as they are or, for added flavor, toast them in a dry skillet over medium heat for 5-7 minutes, stirring occasionally until they become fragrant.
4. Optionally, sprinkle a pinch of salt or your favorite seasoning on the walnuts for extra taste.
5. Let the toasted walnuts cool before serving.
6. Walnuts can be enjoyed on their own or added to salads, yogurt, or as a topping for desserts.
7. Grab a handful of walnuts for a nutritious and satisfying snack, rich in healthy fats and antioxidants!

Dinner: Baked cod with quinoa and roasted asparagus

Ingredients:

For Baked Cod:

- 4 cod fillets
- 2 tablespoons olive oil
- 1 lemon, juiced
- 2 cloves garlic, minced
- 1 teaspoon dried oregano
- Salt and black pepper to taste
- Lemon slices for garnish (optional)

For Quinoa:

- 1 cup quinoa, rinsed
- 2 cups water or vegetable broth

- Salt to taste

For Roasted Asparagus:

- 1 bunch asparagus, trimmed
- 2 tablespoons olive oil
- Salt and black pepper to taste

Instructions:

For Baked Cod:

1. Preheat the oven to 400°F (200°C).
2. In a small bowl, mix olive oil, lemon juice, minced garlic, dried oregano, salt, and black pepper.
3. Place cod fillets in a baking dish. Pour the marinade over the cod, ensuring each fillet is coated.
4. Optionally, place lemon slices on top of each cod fillet.
5. Bake in the preheated oven for 15-20 minutes or until the cod is cooked through and flakes easily with a fork.

For Quinoa:

1. In a saucepan, combine rinsed quinoa and water or vegetable broth. Add salt to taste.
2. Bring to a boil, then reduce heat to low, cover, and simmer for 15-20 minutes or until quinoa is cooked and liquid is absorbed. Fluff with a fork.

For Roasted Asparagus:

1. Preheat the oven to 400°F (200°C).
2. Toss trimmed asparagus with olive oil, salt, and black pepper.
3. Spread the asparagus on a baking sheet in a single layer.
4. Roast in the preheated oven for about 10-12 minutes or until the asparagus is tender but still crisp.

To Serve:

1. Plate a portion of cooked quinoa.
2. Top with baked cod fillets.

3. Serve alongside roasted asparagus.

4. Enjoy this Baked Cod with Quinoa and Roasted Asparagus for a flavorful and well-balanced dinner!

Day 7:

Breakfast: Smoothie with berries, kale, and protein powder

Ingredients:

- 1 cup mixed berries (strawberries, blueberries, raspberries)
- 1 cup kale leaves, stems removed
- 1 scoop protein powder (vanilla or berry-flavored)
- 1/2 banana
- 1 cup almond milk (or your preferred milk)
- Ice cubes (optional)

Instructions:

1. Wash the berries and kale leaves thoroughly.

2. In a blender, combine mixed berries, kale leaves, protein powder, half a banana, and almond milk.

3. Optionally, add ice cubes for a colder smoothie.

4. Blend all the ingredients until smooth and creamy.

5. Taste the smoothie and adjust the sweetness by adding more bananas if needed.

6. Pour the Berry, Kale, and Protein Smoothie into a glass.

7. Optionally, garnish with a few fresh berries on top.

8. Enjoy this nutrient-packed and delicious smoothie as a wholesome breakfast to kickstart your day!

Snack: Apple slices with cheese

Ingredients:

- Fresh apples

- Cheese of your choice (cheddar, gouda, or brie work well)
- Optional: Nut butter, honey, or nuts for topping

Instructions:

1. Wash and slice fresh apples into thin rounds or wedges.
2. Arrange the apple slices on a plate or serving tray.
3. Cut the cheese into small pieces or thin slices.
4. Place a piece of cheese on each apple slice.
5. Optional: Drizzle a small amount of honey or spread a thin layer of nut butter on top of the cheese for added flavor.
6. If you like, sprinkle chopped nuts over the apple slices for extra crunch.
7. Enjoy the Apple Slices with Cheese as a delicious and balanced snack, combining the sweetness of apples with the savory goodness of cheese!

Lunch: Shrimp and vegetable stir-fry with brown rice

Ingredients:

For Shrimp and Vegetable Stir-Fry:

- 1 pound (about 450g) shrimp, peeled and deveined
- 2 cups mixed vegetables (broccoli, bell peppers, snap peas, carrots), chopped
- 3 cloves garlic, minced
- 1 tablespoon ginger, grated
- 2 tablespoons soy sauce
- 1 tablespoon oyster sauce
- 1 tablespoon hoisin sauce
- 1 tablespoon cornstarch
- 2 tablespoons vegetable oil
- Green onions, sliced for garnish

For Brown Rice:

- 1 cup brown rice
- 2 cups water

- Salt to taste

Instructions:

For Brown Rice:

1. In a saucepan, combine brown rice, water, and a pinch of salt.
2. Bring to a boil, then reduce heat to low, cover, and simmer for 45-50 minutes or until rice is cooked and water is absorbed.
3. Fluff the brown rice with a fork.

For Shrimp and Vegetable Stir-Fry:

1. In a bowl, mix soy sauce, oyster sauce, hoisin sauce, and cornstarch.
2. Add peeled and deveined shrimp to the marinade and let them marinate for at least 15 minutes.
3. Heat vegetable oil in a wok or large skillet over high heat.
4. Add minced garlic and grated ginger to the wok, stir-frying for about 30 seconds until fragrant.
5. Add the marinated shrimp to the wok and stir-fry for 2-3 minutes or until they turn pink and opaque. Remove shrimp from the wok and set aside.
6. In the same wok, add a bit more oil if needed and stir-fry the mixed vegetables until they are crisp-tender.
7. Return the cooked shrimp to the wok and pour the sauce over the shrimp and vegetables. Toss everything together until well coated and heated through.
8. Garnish the Shrimp and Vegetable Stir-Fry with sliced green onions.
9. Serve the stir-fry over a bed of brown rice.
10. Enjoy this delicious and healthy Shrimp and Vegetable Stir-Fry with Brown Rice for a satisfying lunch!

Snack: Yogurt with sliced kiwi

Ingredients:

- Greek yogurt (or your preferred yogurt)
- Fresh kiwi, peeled and sliced

- Honey (optional, for drizzling)

Instructions:

1. Spoon Greek yogurt into a bowl or a serving dish.
2. Peel and slice fresh kiwi.
3. Arrange the sliced kiwi on top of the yogurt.
4. Optional: Drizzle honey over the yogurt and kiwi for added sweetness.
5. Serve the Yogurt with Sliced Kiwi as a refreshing and nutritious snack.
6. Enjoy the combination of creamy yogurt and the vibrant, tangy flavor of fresh kiwi!

Dinner: Beef and broccoli stir-fry with cauliflower rice

Ingredients:

For Beef and Broccoli Stir-Fry:

- 1 pound (about 450g) beef sirloin or flank steak, thinly sliced
- 4 cups broccoli florets
- 3 tablespoons soy sauce
- 1 tablespoon oyster sauce
- 1 tablespoon hoisin sauce
- 2 tablespoons cornstarch
- 2 tablespoons vegetable oil
- 3 cloves garlic, minced
- 1 tablespoon ginger, grated
- Sesame seeds for garnish (optional)
- Green onions, sliced for garnish

For Cauliflower Rice:

- 1 large head of cauliflower, grated or processed into rice-like texture
- 2 tablespoons vegetable oil
- Salt and black pepper to taste

Instructions:

For Beef and Broccoli Stir-Fry:

1. In a bowl, mix soy sauce, oyster sauce, hoisin sauce, and cornstarch.
2. Add thinly sliced beef to the marinade and let it marinate for at least 15 minutes.
3. Heat vegetable oil in a wok or large skillet over high heat.
4. Add minced garlic and grated ginger to the wok, stir-frying for about 30 seconds until fragrant.
5. Add the marinated beef to the wok and stir-fry for 2-3 minutes or until it's browned and cooked to your liking. Remove the beef from the wok and set aside.
6. In the same wok, add a bit more oil if needed and stir-fry broccoli florets until they are crisp-tender.
7. Return the cooked beef to the wok and pour the sauce over the beef and broccoli. Toss everything together until well coated and heated through.
8. Garnish the Beef and Broccoli Stir-Fry with sesame seeds and sliced green onions.

For Cauliflower Rice:

1. Grate or process the cauliflower into rice-like texture.
2. Heat vegetable oil in a large skillet over medium heat.
3. Add the cauliflower rice to the skillet and cook for 5-7 minutes, stirring occasionally, until it's tender but not mushy.
4. Season the cauliflower rice with salt and black pepper to taste.

To Serve:

1. Plate a portion of cauliflower rice.
2. Top with the Beef and Broccoli Stir-Fry.
3. Enjoy this flavorful and low-carb Beef and Broccoli Stir-Fry with Cauliflower Rice for a satisfying dinner!

ADAPTING TRADITIONAL RECIPES TO BLOOD TYPE O POSITIVE

1. Choose lean protein sources, like poultry, fish, and lean beef. Avoid processed meats and high-fat cuts.

2. Vegetables such as spinach, kale, and broccoli are excellent for blood type O positive persons.

3. Replace saturated fats with healthy alternatives such as olive, avocado, or nut oils.

4. Choose whole grains, such as quinoa, brown rice, and millet, over refined grains for a blood type O positive diet.

5. For those with blood type O, it is recommended to limit dairy consumption and opt for goat or sheep milk products.

6. Fruits such as berries, cherries, and plums are ideal for blood type O positive persons.

7. Experiment with Herbs & Spices: Use ginger, garlic, and turmeric to add flavor without excessive salt.

8. Reduce wheat-based items by switching to spelt or rice-based alternatives.

9. To preserve nutrients, choose cooking methods such as grilling, baking, or steaming instead of frying.

10. Customize recipes to meet individual tastes and dietary demands, while adhering to general rules for blood type O positives.

11. To stay hydrated, choose herbal teas and water with lemon instead of sugary drinks.

SHOPPING LIST FOR BLOOD TYPE O POSITIVE DIET

Proteins:

- Chicken breast
- Turkey
- Lean beef
- Lamb
- Salmon
- Cod
- Shrimp

Vegetables:

- Spinach
- Kale
- Broccoli
- Brussels sprouts
- Sweet potatoes
- Zucchini
- Onions

Fruits:

- Berries (blueberries, strawberries)
- Cherries
- Plums
- Pineapple
- Apples
- Mangoes
- Kiwi

Grains:

- Quinoa
- Brown rice
- Millet
- Spelt
- Oatmeal (if well-tolerated)

Dairy:

- Goat cheese
- Sheep milk products (if included in the diet)

Fats and Oils:

- Olive oil
- Avocado oil
- Almond butter

Nuts and Seeds:

- Almonds
- Walnuts
- Pumpkin seeds

Herbs and Spices:

- Ginger
- Garlic
- Turmeric
- Basil
- Rosemary

Beverages:

- Green tea
- Herbal teas
- Water with lemon

Miscellaneous:

- Eggs
- Fresh herbs (cilantro, parsley)
- Natural sweeteners (honey, maple syrup - in moderation)
- Fresh vegetables for salads (cucumbers, tomatoes)

COOKING TIPS FOR BLOOD TYPE O POSITIVE

1. Prioritize lean proteins.

   Choose lean protein sources such as chicken, fish, and lean cuts of meat. Trim any visible fat before cooking.

2. Embrace grilling and baking.

   Instead of frying, choose to grill, bake, or steam. These strategies aid in nutrient retention while avoiding excessive additional fats.

3. Experiment with herbs and spices.

   Instead of using excessive salt or high-sodium condiments, add flavor using herbs and spices such as ginger, garlic, and turmeric.

4. Incorporate Beneficial Vegetables.

    Incorporate veggies such as spinach, kale, and broccoli into your meals to boost nutritious content.

5. Choose whole grains.

    For prolonged energy, choose whole grains such as quinoa, brown rice, and spelt.

6. Investigate Alternative Flours:

    To eliminate wheat-based items, try baking using alternatives such as almond or spelt flour.

7. Mindful Dairy Choices:

    When introducing dairy, use goat or sheep milk products, as these are frequently better accepted.

8. Use Healthy Fats:

    Cook with healthy fats like olive oil, avocado oil, and almonds.

9. Limit processed foods.

    Reduce your intake of processed and packaged foods, which may include ingredients that are incompatible with blood type O.

10. Prepare Balanced Meals.

    To improve overall nutrition, prepare balanced meals with a variety of proteins, veggies, and healthy fats.

11. Stay hydrated:

    Hydrate with water or herbal teas and avoid sugary drinks.